Psychiatry at a Glance

Psychiatry at a Glance

Cornelius Katona

Honorary Professor, Department of Mental and Health Sciences, University College London; Honorary Consultant Psychiatrist, Kent and Medway NHS and Social Care Partnership Trust

Claudia Cooper

Senior Lecturer in Old Age Psychiatry, University College London; Honorary Consultant Psychiatrist, Camden and Islington Foundation Trust

Mary Robertson

Emeritus Professor in Neuropsychiatry, University College London; Visiting Professor and Honorary Consultant, St George's Hospital and Medical School London

Fourth edition

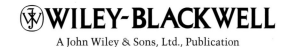
A John Wiley & Sons, Ltd., Publication

This edition first published 2008, © 1995, 2000, 2005 by Cornelius Katona, Claudia Cooper, Mary Robertson

Blackwell Publishing was acquired by John Wiley & Sons in February 2007. Blackwell's publishing program has been merged with Wiley's global Scientific, Technical and Medical business to form Wiley-Blackwell.

Registered office: John Wiley & Sons Ltd, The Atrium, Southern Gate, Chichester, West Sussex, PO19 8SQ, UK

Editorial offices: 9600 Garsington Road, Oxford, OX4 2DQ, UK
    The Atrium, Southern Gate, Chichester, West Sussex, PO19 8SQ, UK
    111 River Street, Hoboken, NJ 07030-5774, USA

For details of our global editorial offices, for customer services and for information about how to apply for permission to reuse the copyright material in this book please see our website at www.wiley.com/wiley-blackwell

Library of Congress Cataloging-in-Publication Data
Katona, C. L. E. (Cornelius L. E.), 1954–
   Psychiatry at a glance / Cornelius Katona, Mary Robertson, Claudia Cooper. – 4th ed.
     p. ; cm. – (At a glance series)
   Includes bibliographical references and index.
   ISBN 978-1-4051-8117-4 (pbk. : alk. paper)
   1. Psychiatry. I. Robertson, Mary M. II. Cooper, Claudia. III. Title IV. Series: At a glance series (Oxford, England)
   [DNLM: 1. Mental Disorders. 2. Mental Disorders–therapy. 3. Psychiatry. WM 140 K19p 2008]

   RC454.K366 2008
   616.89–dc22

                            2008023800

ISBN: 978-1-4051-8117-4

A catalogue record for this book is available from the British Library.

Set in 9 on 11.5 pt Times by SNP Best-set Typesetter Ltd., Hong Kong
Printed in Singapore by Utopia Press Pte Ltd

1 2008

Commissioning Editor: Elizabeth Johnston
Development Editor: Laura Murphy
Editorial Assistant: Madeleine Hurd
Production Controller: Debbie Wyer

Contents

Preface

We are delighted that demand for *Psychiatry at a Glance* continues. This, and the specific feedback we receive, suggest that medical students and others continue to need a short summary of core psychiatric knowledge and skills. As before, though the book is intended primarily for a medical student readership, we think it will be useful to qualified doctors preparing for specialist exams, to psychology students and trainees, and to nurses and other allied health professionals. We are very much aware of recent changes to the content and (more strikingly) to the assessment methods used by medical and other health schools. We have therefore made more substantial changes in this fourth edition than in any previous revision. In particular, as well as thorough review of all existing text and diagrammatic content, we have added a chapter on social exclusion (chapter 24) and described current and forthcoming mental health and capacity legislation across the four UK jurisdictions (chapters 40–42). We have enlarged the content of the psychiatric history and the mental state examination, enabling division into two chapters (chapters 1–2). Since the book is aimed at a predominantly European readership, we have concentrated on describing the World Health Organization diagnostic criteria and categories (ICD 10); we have, however, mentioned the American Psychiatric Association criteria (DSM-IV-TR) where these are relevant. The content on treatments has been very substantially enlarged, necessitating four rather than two chapters (chapters 34–37). We have added a Glossary to help readers unfamiliar with specialist psychiatric terminology and have fully updated the Further Reading section, focusing on up-to-date reviews. We have increased the focus on preparation for exams with an enlarged chapter on self-assessment to include Extended Matching Questions (EMQs) as well as expanding the chapter on preparing for clinical examinations (chapter 43) to help students prepare for the OSCE component, which is now ubiquitous.

This fourth edition has three authors: Professors Cornelius Katona and Mary Robertson have been very fortunate in recruiting Dr Claudia Cooper who was the best trainee either of them has had the pleasure of working with and who has both the academic and writing skills to ensure that the new edition is fully up-to-date, relevant to current practice and intelligible. We have all three found the experience of collaborating on this new edition to be both intellectually stimulating and highly enjoyable.

As before, we have obtained feedback on the content of each chapter both from recently qualified doctors and from experts in the field. We are therefore pleased to have this opportunity to thank our colleagues for assisting us in taking the *Psychiatry at a Glance* project forward. These include Professors Abou-Saleh, Bhui, Casey, Christodoulou, Eapen, Fineberg, King, Kohen, Livingston, Rihmer, Schmidt and Scott and Doctors Baldwin, Bass, Bird, Bishop, Black, Cookson, Cotton, Cutinha, Davidson, Dein, Dutton, Hashmi, Hassiotis, Khalifeh, Killaspy, Lydall, Mijovic, Owens, Paradise, Previtera, Regan, Rickards, Ring, Rodda, Shah, Shergill, Tandy, Taylor, Thinn, Turjanski, Walker, Yacoub, Young and de Zulueta. Responsibility for any errors or inaccuracies remains, of course, entirely ours.

Philippa Katona and John Ludgate have remained stalwart supporters of *Psychiatry at a Glance*, for which we are, as ever, extremely grateful. We are also grateful to Mike Carless for his patience and support.

Cornelius Katona
Claudia Cooper
Mary Robertson

1 The psychiatric history

Psychiatric history	Case example
Introduction and presenting complaint	**Introduction and presenting complaint:** Mr John Smith is a 36 year old Caucasian gentleman, who was admitted to Florence Ward three days ago, after police detained him on Section 136 acting bizarrely in the street. He was assessed in A+E and placed on a Section 2. His main concern is that his neighbours are plotting to kill him.
History of Presenting complaint	**History of presenting complaint:** Mr Smith reports that he last felt free from worry four months ago. Since this time, after witnessing the man next door staring at him when he was out, he has become increasingly concerned about the activities of this neighbour and his wife. He believes they are intercepting his mail, and have a machine to do this so noone can tell letters have been opened. He often sees red cars outside which he thinks are used by these neighbours to monitor his movements. He smelt a "strange gas" in the flat recently and concluded they had pumped this through holes in the ceiling. In the last week he reports things have escalated and after an altercation on the street three days ago in which he accused these neighbours of pumping gas into his flat, he realised that they want to kill him. He believes they want to force him to leave the house so they can purchase the property for their expanding family. He denied feeling low in mood, and is more angry about the situation. He cannot rule out the possibility he might defend himself if he felt threatened by the neighbours, but denies specific plans to retaliate against the perceived persecution. He denies hearing the neighbours or others talking about him or feeling that they can control him or his thoughts. He has been sleeping poorly due to worrying about the situation. His appetite is good.
Past Psychiatric history	**Past psychiatric history:** Mr Smith has seen a psychiatrist once before, aged 8, when he was diagnosed with "emotional problems". His GP diagnosed depression when he was 24, and prescribed Fluoxetine which he never took. He believes he was depressed for a couple of years in his mid-twenties but denies mental health problems since then. No previous psychiatric admissions. He has never taken medication for mental illness.
Past medical/surgical history	**Past medical/surgical history:** Mild asthma. Nil else of note.
Drug History and Allergies	**Drug history and allergies:** No current medication. No known allergies.
Family history	**Family history:** His father died from lung cancer aged 60 when Mr Smith was 28. His mother and brother (eight years younger) live near by. Both are well, in regular contact and supportive. No known family psychiatric history.
Personal history	**Personal history**
Early life and development	**Early life and development:** Mr Smith was born by Normal Vaginal Delivery, with no known complications. There was no developmental delay. The family lived in the same house in Doncaster throughout his childhood. His father was a computer salesman, and his mother was a housewife. He believes his parents were happily married, and there were no financial problems at home. At the age of 6 his maternal grandmother and grandfather died in a car crash. He remembers this as an unhappy time, and recalls being left on his own to play for hours on end. Two years later his brother was born and the years after this were happier. He denies mental or physical abuse.
Educational history	**Educational history:** Mr Smith left school at 16 with 5 GCE's. He had good friends from school. He was often in trouble with his teachers, was suspended once for cheating in an exam, but was never expelled.
Occupational history	**Occupational history:** After leaving school he worked in the family plumbing business for a few years, before leaving to train as a mechanic. He completed his training and has worked as a mechanic since this time. He has never been sacked, and has been in his current job for three years, which is his longest period of consecutive employment; he has a good relationship with his employer. He has been on sick leave for the last two weeks due to stress.
Relationship history	**Relationship history:** Happily married for 10 years. He has one daughter, aged 5 who is well.
Substance use	**Substance use:** Mr Smith drinks 30 units of alcohol a week, mainly wine in the evenings. There is no history of alcohol dependence. He has used cannabis regularly in the past (aged 16-28) but no illicit drug use since this time.
Forensic history	**Forensic history:** One conviction for driving without due care in 1990, for which he received a fine. No other arrests or convictions reported.
Social history	**Social history:** Mr Smith owns his three bedroom detached house. He has friends from his cycling club who he usually sees weekly, although not for the past month. He works fulltime in a garage. No current financial difficulties.
Premorbid personality	**Premorbid personality:** He described himself as being a sociable, calm person who thought the best of people and didn't tend to get into disputes with others prior to his current difficulties. He is a keen cyclist and member of a local cycling club, and attends church weekly. He obtains comfort from this and has some friends with whom he socializes at parish functions.

Informant history

Taking a psychiatric history and assessing the mental state (discussed in Chapter 2) are undertaken together in the *psychiatric interview*. As well as systematically obtaining this information, it is crucial to establish and maintain a rapport with the patient. In this chapter and the next, we present a format for written documentation; greater flexibility is clearly required during the actual interview.

Introduction and presenting complaint

Begin your history with a brief *introduction*, including the patient's name, age, occupation, ethnic origin, circumstances of referral and presenting *complaint* (in the patient's own words).

History of the present illness

When did the problem begin, or if the person has a longstanding, relapsing, remitting illness, when were they last well? Ask about perceived precipitating factors, the effect on personal relationships and their capacity to work. What does the patient think might have caused the illness as a whole or this relapse/recurrence, and what makes it better or worse?

Especially in psychosis, the patient's view of events might differ from those of their family, friends or other collateral sources. In this case, you can record their account, followed by any collateral information available.

Depending on the presenting complaint, you will need to ask follow-up questions about other symptoms to help you make a diagnosis. Your questions should be guided by the diagnostic criteria for the individual disorders (discussed in later chapters). For example, if the patient describes feeling anxious, you would ask questions to establish if the anxiety is situational and if panic attacks occur. You should usually enquire about mood, sleep and appetite, even if they appear normal, and whether there are risks to self or others (see Chapters 4 and 5).

Previous psychiatric history

Give dates of illnesses, symptoms, diagnoses, treatments, hospitalizations, including whether they have been treated under compulsory admission or treatment.

Past medical/surgical history
Drug history and allergies

Include psychotropic medications which the person has received previously, their dosage and duration, and whether or not they helped. The patient or family may not have this information and it may be necessary to obtain it from the patient's GP or hospital notes.

Family history

Note parents' and siblings' ages, occupations, physical and mental health, and quality of their relationship with the patient. If a relative is deceased, note the cause of death and the patient's age at the time of death and their reaction to that death (see Chapter 10). Ask about family history of psychiatric illness ('nervous breakdowns'), suicide, drug and /or alcohol abuse, forensic encounters and medical illnesses.

Personal history
Early life and development

Include details of the pregnancy and birth (especially complications), any serious illnesses, bereavements, emotional, physical or sexual abuse, separations in childhood or developmental delays. Describe the childhood home environment (note atmosphere, any deprivation).

Educational history

Include details of school, academic achievements, relationships with peers (did they have any friends?) and conduct (whether suspended or expelled). Bullying and school refusal or truancy should be explored.

Occupational history

List job titles and duration, reasons for change, work satisfaction and relationships with colleagues. The longest duration of continuous employment is a good indicator of pre-morbid functioning.

Relationship history

Document details of relationships and marriages (duration, details of partner, children, abuse); sexual practices, difficulties and orientation; in the case of women, menstrual pattern, contraception, miscarriages, stillbirths and any termination(s) of pregnancy. Those who are in a long-term relationship should be asked about the support they receive from their partner and the quality of the relationship – whether there is good communication, aggression (physical or verbal), jealousy or infidelity.

Substance use

Alcohol, drug (prescribed and recreational) and tobacco consumption.

Forensic history

Note any arrests, whether they resulted in conviction and whether they were for violent offences. Report any periods of imprisonment, for what they were imprisoned and the length of time served.

Social history

Describe current accommodation, occupation, financial details and daily activities.

Premorbid personality

A description of the patient's character and attitudes before they became unwell (e.g. character, social relations). You could ask the patient how they would describe themselves before their current difficulties and how their friends would describe them; what they enjoy doing; how they cope with adversity; whether they practise any religion and if they get comfort from this, or details of social contacts with religious or other groups/organisations.

2 The mental state examination

Mental state examination		Example
Appearance and behaviour		*Appearance and behaviour*: Mr Smith was a thin gentleman, appropriately dressed in casual clothes, with no evidence of poor personal hygiene or abnormal movements; he was not objectively hallucinating. He was polite, appropriate in behaviour, maintained good eye contact, and although it was initially difficult to establish a rapport, this improved throughout the interview.
Speech and thought form		*Speech*: normal in tone, rate and volume. Relevant and coherent, with no evidence of formal thought disorder.
Tone	Flight of ideas	
Rate	Loosening of associations	
Volume		
Mood (subjective and objective)		*Mood*: subjectively "fine", objectively euthymic.
Affect (observed)		*Affect*: suspicious at times, particularly when discussing treatment; reactive.
Thought content		*Thoughts*: persecutory delusions and delusions of reference elicited. Could not "rule out" retaliating against neighbour, but no current thoughts, plans or intent to harm neighbour, self or anyone else. No evidence of depressive cognitions or anxiety symptoms. No suicidal ideation.
Depressive/anxious cognitions	Overvalued ideas	
	Ideas of reference	
Preoccupations	Delusions	
Obsessions	Suicidal/homicidal	
Perception		*Perception*: no abnormality detected
Hallucinations	Pseudo-hallucinations	
Illusions		
Cognition		*Cognition*: alert, orientated to time, place and person. No impairment of concentration or memory noted during interview.
Consciousness	Orientation	
Attention/concentration	Intelligence	
Memory	Executive function	
Insight		*Insight*: Patient believes he is stressed; he is aware that others think he has a psychotic illness but he disagrees with this. He does not want to receive any treatment and does not think he needs to be in hospital. He would be willing to see a counsellor for stress.

Physical examination

This chapter describes the information that should be reported in the mental state examination.

Appearance and behaviour

Describe general health, build, whether of good personal hygiene and tidily dressed/well-kempt; any unusual clothing or striking physical features; manner, rapport, eye contact, degree of cooperation, facial expression, posture, whether responding to hallucinations. Also note any unusual tattoos, piercings, venepuncture sites or lacerations (especially on the forearm). Motor activity may be excessive (psychomotor agitation) or decreased (psychomotor retardation).

Look for extrapyramidal symptoms or side-effects of antipsychotic medication. These include Parkinsonian symptoms such as tremor and bradykinesia (slowness of movement), akathisia (restlessness); tardive dyskinesia (movements most often affecting the mouth, lips and tongue [e.g. rolling the tongue or licking the lips]) and dystonia (muscular spasm causing abnormal face and body movement or posture). Other abnormal movements include tics, chorea, stereotypy (repetitive, purposeless movements [e.g. rocking in people with severe learning disability]), mannerisms (goal-directed, understandable movements [e.g. saluting]); and gait abnormality.

Speech

Describe tone (variation in pitch; reduced sometimes in depression), rate (speed) and volume (quantity). In pressure of speech, rate and volume are increased and speech may be uninterruptible. In depression, tone, rate and volume are often decreased, and there may be poverty of thought.

'Normal' speech can be described as 'spontaneous, logical, relevant and coherent'; 'circumstantial' speech is discursive and takes a long time to get to the point. Note any perseveration (repeating words or topics) and abnormal words (neologisms, e.g. headshoe to mean hat).

Thought form

This may be deduced where connections between statements are difficult to follow. In flight of ideas there is an abnormal connection between statements based on a rhyme or pun rather than meaning (e.g. 'You come in here swinging your stethoscope, telling me about my horoscope'). Speech is often pressured. In 'loosening of associations' there is no discernible link between statements: 'The tablets are red, I think climate change is a concern, what do you want with the piano?'

Give verbatim examples if thought form is abnormal. The patient's subjective experience of thought may be abnormal as in thought block (thoughts disappear: 'my mind goes blank').

Mood and affect

Abnormalities are the commonest symptoms of psychiatric disorder, but also occur in physical illness and in healthy people.

Mood is the underlying emotion; report subjective mood (in patient's own words) and objective mood (described as dysthymic, euthymic or elated/hyperthymic).

Affect is the observed (and often more transient) external manifestation of emotion. Mood has been compared to climate and affect to weather. Abnormalities of affect include being blunted/unreactive (lacking normal emotional responses); conventionally, this affect is often described as blunted if resulting from negative symptoms of schizophrenia, and unreactive in depression; labile (excessively changeable); irritable (which may occur in mania, depression); perplexed; suspicious; or incongruous (grossly out of tune with subjects being discussed, e.g. laughing about bereavement). Where no abnormality is detected affect is reactive (appropriate response to emotional cues).

Disorders of thought content

Report here any negative (depressed) cognitions of guilt, hopelessness, worthlessness or low self-esteem. Ruminations (persistent preoccupations) may occur in depression or anxiety.

Report any subjective anxiety and main subject of worries, obsessional ideas (Chapter 12) and phobias (Chapter 11). Record the presence and frequency of any panic attacks during the interview.

Depersonalization is the unpleasant experience of subjective change, feeling detached, unreal, empty within, unable to feel emotion, watching oneself from the outside ('It feels as if I am cut off by a pane of glass'). Derealization is the experience of the world or people in it seeming lifeless ('as if all in the world is made out of cardboard'). Depersonalization and derealization are not psychotic phenomena, although some erroneously describe them as such.

Abnormal beliefs include overvalued ideas (an acceptable, comprehensible idea pursued by the patient beyond the bounds of reason and to an extent that causes distress to the patient or those around him or her). An example of this would be an intense but non-delusional feeling of guilty responsibility following bereavement. Ideas of reference are thoughts that other people are looking at or talking about the patient, not held with delusional intensity. Delusions are fixed, false, firmly held beliefs out of keeping with the patient's culture which are unaltered by evidence to the contrary.

Here are some types of delusions, and questions you might ask to elicit them (see also Chapter 6).

Delusion type:	Content	Example question
Persecutory	Someone or something is interfering with the person in a malicious/destructive way	Do you worry that people are against you or trying to harm you?
Grandiose	Being famous, having supernatural powers or enormous wealth	Do you have any exceptional abilities or talents?
Of reference	Actions of other people, events, media etc. are referring to the person or communicating a message	Have you heard people talking about you? Have you heard things on the TV or radio you think are about you?
Thought insertion/withdrawal/broadcast	Thoughts can be controlled by an outside influence: inserted, withdrawn or broadcast to others	Do you feel your thoughts are being interfered with or controlled? Are they known to others, e.g. through telepathy?
Passivity	Actions, feelings or impulses can be controlled or interfered with by outside influence	Do you feel another person can control what you do directly, as if pulling puppet strings?

Suicidal ideation, should be recorded, and whether the patient intends to act on these thoughts or has a plan about how he or she would do so.

Perception

Describe here any illusions (distortions of perception of an external stimulus, e.g. interpreting a curtain cord as a snake). Illusions can occur in healthy people. Hallucinations (perceptions in the absence of an external stimulus which are experienced both as true and as coming from the outside world); and pseudo-hallucinations (internal perceptions with preserved insight). Hallucinations can occur in any sensory modality, although auditory and visual are commonest. Some auditory hallucinations occur in normal individuals when falling asleep (hypnagogic) or on waking (hypnopompic).

Cognition

Note at least level of consciousness, memory (long- and short-term, immediate recall), orientation in time (day, date, time), place, person; attention and concentration. In people over 65 or who have any evidence of cognitive impairment, this section should be extended to include formal testing of memory, orientation, dyspraxia, agnosia, receptive and expressive dysphasia and executive functioning (e.g. by completing a Mini-Mental State Examination [MMSE] with additional tests of frontal lobe function). These could include estimating (e.g. approximate the height of a local landmark); abstract reasoning (ask how many camels in Belgium – answer 1–50); tests of verbal fluency (can they think of at least 15 words beginning with each of the letters F, A and S in a minute?) and proverb interpretation.

Insight

Record here the patient's understanding of their condition and its cause as well as their willingness to accept treatment.

Physical examination

This should focus on identifying (or excluding) conditions of which a suspicion has been raised in the history and mental state examination and those with a known association with psychiatric illness.

3 Diagnosis and classification in psychiatry

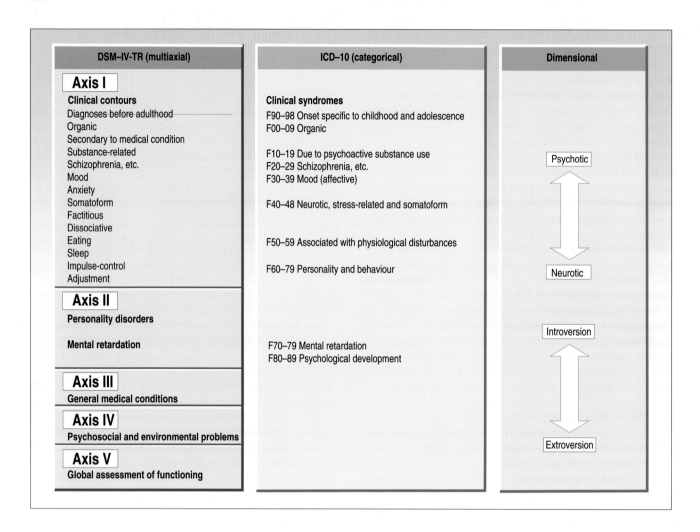

History

Diagnoses and classifications in psychiatry have undergone tremendous changes in the last 60 years. Before the 1950s, diagnoses were not only unreliable, but even had meanings that varied considerably across the world. By the end of that decade, 'antipsychiatrists', including R. D. Laing and Thomas Szasz, had started to suggest that diagnoses and classification in psychiatry should be abandoned, together with the concept of mental illness. In the 1960s, the World Health Organization (WHO) instigated a world-wide programme (of more than 30 countries) aimed at improving diagnosis and classification of mental disorders, fostering research into reliability of diagnosis and classification. The mental health section of the International Classification of Diseases (ICD) has subsequently been revised several times and is currently in its 10th edition (ICD-10). The American Psychiatric Association developed its own classificatory system, the Diagnostic and Statistical Manual of Mental Disorders (DSM); the current classification, DSM-IV-TR, was published in 2000.

The concept of mental illness

In general medicine, a distinction is made between 'disease' (objective physical pathology and known aetiology) and 'illness' (subjective distress). Psychiatric conditions without organic cause should not therefore be considered 'diseases' since in many there is no demonstrable pathology. The advent of new techniques (e.g. neuroimaging) may, however, result in the emergence of definable psychiatric diseases.

The concept of mental 'illness' is useful in defining a level of subjective distress greater in severity and/or duration than occurs in normal human experience. In addition, the legislation in many countries requires psychiatrists to diagnose defined 'mental illness' when certifying the need for compulsory hospital treatment and in forensic (legal) psychiatry.

Aims and purposes

The purpose of classification in psychiatry, as in general medicine, is first, to identify groups of patients who are similar in their clinical features, course of disease, outcome and response to treatment, thus not only aiding individual clinical management, but also providing patterns of treatment response and prognosis, which can be extrapolated to future patients. A second purpose is to facilitate communication between professionals and their research into the aetiology, prevention and treatment of psychiatric conditions. A third aim of classification is to improve the *reliability* (reproducibility among different settings) and *validity*

 Psychiatry at a Glance, 4e. By C. Katona, C. Cooper and M. Robertson. Published 2008 Blackwell Publishing. ISBN: 978-1-4501-8117-4

(correctness) of diagnoses. Validity is more difficult to confirm, but attempts have been made, including the examination of consistency of symptom patterns (statistical procedures such as cluster analysis facilitate this) and demonstration of consistent treatment responses, long-term prognoses, genetic and biological correlates.

Discriminating symptoms occur commonly in a defined syndrome, but rarely in other syndromes (e.g. thought broadcast/schizophrenia [see Chapter 6]). *Characteristic symptoms* occur frequently in the defined syndrome but also occur in other syndromes (e.g. depressed mood, which though common in depressive illness also occurs in schizophrenia, alcoholism, etc.). *Operational definitions* specify precise inclusion and exclusion criteria.

Types of classification

Traditionally, mental disorder is differentiated into: *mental retardation* (learning disability, in which features of the disorder have been present from birth or an early age); *personality disorder* (usually developing through childhood or adolescence and clearly evident from early adulthood with no period of normal adult functioning); *mental illness* (where there is an identifiable onset of illness preceded by normal functioning); *adjustment disorder* (less severe than mental illness, occurring in relation to stressful events or changed circumstances); *disorders of childhood and adolescence; and other disorders* (those that do not fit into any other group, including behavioural disorders and substance misuse).

The three main classification systems are categorical, multiaxial and dimensional:

• *Categorical systems* describe a group of entirely discrete conditions which are usually classified hierarchically, so that each patient can receive one main diagnosis: organic psychoses (those with a discernible physical cause [e.g. tumour, drug use]) take precedence over functional psychoses (those where no physical cause can be found) which take precedence over neuroses. The terms *psychosis* (severe mental disturbance characterized by a loss of contact with external reality, delusions, hallucinations and disorganized thinking are often present) and *neurosis* (mental distress in which the ability to distinguish between symptoms originating from patient's own mind and external reality is retained; includes most depressive and anxiety disorders) are widely used and may be regarded as a categorical system.

• *Multiaxial systems* categorize the patient on several axes (each a categorical system). DSM uses a multiaxial system.

• *Dimensional systems* use a continuum rather than categories and have been used mainly to classify personality. For example, Hans Eysenck has proposed three dimensions of personality: introversion/extroversion, neuroticism and psychoticism. A psychotic/neurotic continuum for major mental illness has been suggested by K. E. Kendell.

Systems of classification

The two main current systems of classification (both categorical) are the DSM (American Psychiatric Association) and the ICD (World Health Organization International Classification of Diseases).

DSM-IV-TR is a *multiaxial* system and relies on operational criteria. These state which symptoms must be present for each diagnosis to be made (often quantifying their number and requiring a minimum duration) as well as exclusion criteria. DSM-IV-TR describes a patient's illness on five axes:

Axis I – clinical syndromes and other conditions that may be a focus of clinical attention.

Axis II – personality disorders and mental retardation (the latter classified by severity rather than aetiology).

Axis III – general medical conditions.

Axis IV – psychosocial and environmental problems.

Axis V – the assessor's impression of the patient's global assessment of functioning, on a scale from 100 (excellent functioning) to 0.

ICD-10 is mainly used as a *uniaxial* system, which attempts to standardize diagnoses using descriptive definitions of the syndromes, as well as producing directives on differential diagnosis.

A research supplement to ICD-10 provides operational criteria similar to those of DSM-IV-TR.

ICD-10 and DSM-IV-TR use broadly matching, although not always identical, major diagnostic categories as follows:

1 Disorders Usually First Diagnosed in Infancy, Childhood or Adolescence (which may reflect developmental disorders, discrete illnesses or a combination of the two).

2 Delirium, Dementia, Amnestic and other Cognitive Disorders.

3 Mental Disorders Due to a General Medical Condition not Elsewhere Classified.

4 Psychoactive Substance-related Disorders.

5 Schizophrenia (including Schizotypal, Delusional and other Psychotic Disorders).

6 Mood (affective) Disorders.

7 Anxiety (neurotic) Disorders.

8 Somatoform, Factitious and Dissociative Disorders.

9 Sexual and Identity Disorders.

10 Eating Disorders.

11 Sleep Disorders.

12 Impulse-control Disorders.

13 Adjustment Disorders.

Risk assessment and management in psychiatry

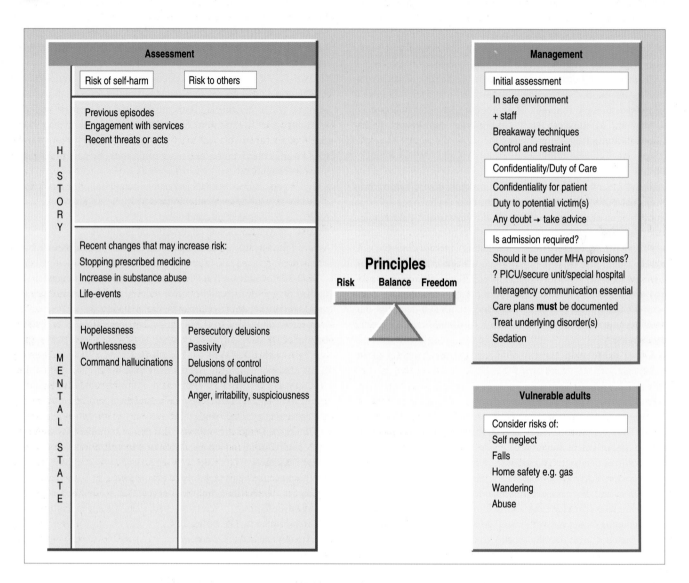

Patients' management should be as unrestrictive and normalizing as possible. Clinicians are required to balance the need to reduce risk as far as possible with the duty to respect patient's rights and freedom; risk cannot be eliminated completely. This continuing process, integral to both hospital and community psychiatry, is termed risk assessment and management.

Risk assessment

All psychiatric patients should have a risk assessment to assess the level of risk they pose to themselves and to others (specific named people or risk of indiscriminate violence). This needs to be reviewed regularly since degree of risk is sensitive to changing circumstances and to a patient's changing mental state. Past behaviour is the best indictor of future behaviour and should be considered in addition to the current history and mental state. History from informants (e.g. family, hostel staff) and a review of case notes and other documentation are critical to ensure all important information is considered.

Initial assessment

Initial assessment of all patients, particularly those already identified as being at high risk, should take place in as safe an environment as possible. The environment in which the patient is being examined or cared for must be assessed and modified to minimize risk. Potential access to harmful agents (firearms, knives, other weapons, incendiary devices, objects that can be used as weapons) should be considered. Where risk is anticipated, one should ensure that senior staff are present where possible. Assessment areas should have appropriate alarm facilities and exit routes.

At the end of the initial assessment, it should be possible to estimate the level of risk in terms of seriousness, specificity, immediacy and potential for rapid change. This should form the basis of a management plan aimed at risk reduction.

Risk of self-harm

In the psychiatric history, ask about current suicidal thoughts ('Have

 Psychiatry at a Glance, 4e. By C. Katona, C. Cooper and M. Robertson. Published 2008 Blackwell Publishing. ISBN: 978-1-4501-8117-4

you thought recently that you want to end your life?'), plans ('Have you thought how you might do this?') and intent ('Do you think that you would actually do this?'). Ask also about anything that prevents the patient acting on their thoughts (e.g. family, religion).

Document previous episodes of deliberate self-harm in detail (circumstances, method and management). Screen for factors predisposing to deliberate self-harm or actual suicide (see Chapter 7). These include a family history of suicide, social isolation and substance misuse. In the mental state, thoughts of hopelessness and worthlessness indicate increased risk; command hallucinations may incite self-harm. Subsequent risk of self-harm is also affected by the likelihood of future engagement with services, so the patient's current intentions and any history of disengagement from services are also relevant.

Risk of harm to others

From the psychiatric interview and case notes, document any history of violence (frequency, severity, nature and most serious resulting harm). Note any history of deliberate fire-setting. Previous episodes of containment (compulsory detention, treatment in special hospital, secure unit, locked ward, prison or police station) are important. Acts or threats of violence or sexually inappropriate behaviour (to family, strangers, staff or other patients) should also be documented. Once again, methods used and resultant injury should be noted. Impulsivity and unpredictability increase risk.

As for self-harm, extent of compliance with previous and current psychiatric treatment and aftercare, alcohol or drug misuse (or any other disinhibiting factors) and extent of social integration are important. Past or current episodes of disengagement from psychiatric follow-up should be noted. Recent stressful life-events, changes in personal circumstances, lack or loss of social support may increase risk, as may recent discontinuation of prescribed drugs or change in use of recreational drugs. More generally, evidence of 'social restlessness' (frequent changes of relationships, work or domicile) indicates increased risk and should be documented. Within the mental state examination (see Chapter 2) key features include expressed violent intentions or threats, irritability, disinhibition, suspiciousness, persecutory delusions (especially with specific person(s) involved), delusions of control or passivity phenomena and command hallucinations.

Risk to children (those referred in their own right or whose parents have a mental illness) should be assessed. Both confidentiality (with regards the patient) and duty to the child must be considered carefully and, if in doubt, advice taken.

Risk of self-neglect and accidental harm

People with mental illness may lack the motivation (e.g. due to severe depression, chronic schizophrenia) or skills (dementia, learning disability) to care for themselves and/or to arrange access to necessary services (e.g. heating, lighting, housing and health care). This can result in serious health risks from malnutrition, failure to access health care or living in squalid conditions.

Falls may occur due to physical frailty, or alcohol or drug intoxication. Self-neglect may also cause risks to others, for example from failure to take adequate safeguards against fire (cigarette-burned bedclothes indicate such a risk) or explosion (from leaving the gas on). When assessing people with dementia, it is important to ask informants about safety while cooking (especially if with gas) and wandering (leaving the house and being unable to find their way home).

Vulnerability to abuse

Abuse is defined as a single or repeated act or lack of appropriate action occurring within any relationship where there is an expectation of trust, which causes harm or distress to a vulnerable person (e.g. older people, people with learning disabilities). People living in institutions may be at particular risk. Abuse also occurs in private homes and this may relate to high levels of stress in family carers. Carers are often themselves subject to such behaviours and this should also be enquired into.

Management

Clinical management of risk involves decisions as to whether admission is necessary, and if so whether this should be under the provisions of the Mental Health Act (Chapters 40–42) and/or to a psychiatric intensive care unit (PICU) or secure unit. Nursing staff in psychiatric units are trained in safe methods of control and restraint of patients, the first stage of which is always to try to manage the situation by 'talking down'. Very occasionally, it is necessary to manage violent and aggressive patients in seclusion for short periods of time to ensure the safety of staff and other patients. All staff working in psychiatry should be trained in 'breakaway' techniques for escaping from violent situations. Level of monitoring should be specified for patients in the community and for those in hospital. Medication may play an important role both in treating any underlying psychiatric disorder and (in patients with high levels of arousal) in inducing sedation or tranquilization (see Chapters 34 and 36). Communication between agencies (particularly Health, Probation and Social Services) is crucial in planning future care in the community of patients at high risk, who are likely to need a high level of supervision that is practical and acceptable. Care plans and their implementation must be negotiated by all involved parties (including the patients themselves, their family and other informal carers), and fully documented.

Breaking confidentiality

Patients have a right to expect that information about them will be held in confidence by their doctors. If, however, doctors are aware of a specific threat to a named individual, they have a duty to ensure that that person is informed. In very rare circumstances, disclosure of patients' information may be justified in the public interest, even if the patient withholds their consent (e.g. if disclosure may assist in the prevention, detection or prosecution of a serious crime). Doctors also have a responsibility to report abuse occurring to children and vulnerable adults (people with dementia, learning disability or others who cannot make decisions about their own welfare) to appropriate agencies (Social Services or, in very serious cases, the police).

5 Suicide and deliberate self-harm

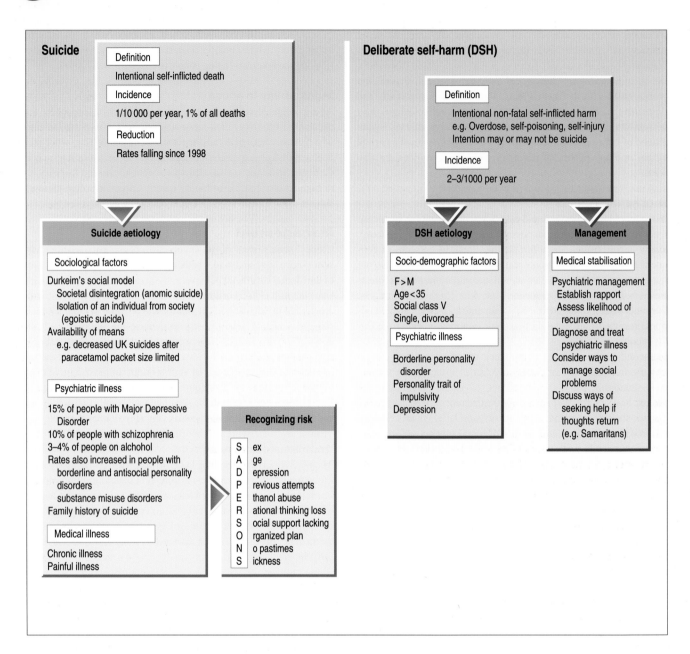

Suicide

| Definition |
Intentional self-inflicted death

| Incidence |
1/10 000 per year, 1% of all deaths

| Reduction |
Rates falling since 1998

Deliberate self-harm (DSH)

| Definition |
Intentional non-fatal self-inflicted harm
e.g. Overdose, self-poisoning, self-injury
Intention may or may not be suicide

| Incidence |
2–3/1000 per year

Suicide aetiology

| Sociological factors |
Durkeim's social model
   Societal disintegration (anomic suicide)
   Isolation of an individual from society
    (egoistic suicide)
Availability of means
   e.g. decreased UK suicides after
   paracetamol packet size limited

| Psychiatric illness |
15% of people with Major Depressive
  Disorder
10% of people with schizophrenia
3–4% of people on alchohol
Rates also increased in people with
  borderline and antisocial personality
  disorders
  substance misuse disorders
Family history of suicide

| Medical illness |
Chronic illness
Painful illness

Recognizing risk

S	ex
A	ge
D	epression
P	revious attempts
E	thanol abuse
R	ational thinking loss
S	ocial support lacking
O	rganized plan
N	o pastimes
S	ickness

DSH aetiology

| Socio-demographic factors |
F > M
Age < 35
Social class V
Single, divorced

| Psychiatric illness |
Borderline personality
  disorder
Personality trait of
  impulsivity
Depression

Management

| Medical stabilisation |
Psychiatric management
  Establish rapport
  Assess likelihood of
   recurrence
Diagnose and treat
  psychiatric illness
Consider ways to
  manage social
  problems
Discuss ways of
  seeking help if
  thoughts return
  (e.g. Samaritans)

The assessment and acute management of deliberate self-harm (DSH) is probably the most critical psychiatric task that doctors face in the early years following qualification. Suicide may be defined as intentional, self-inflicted death; DSH represents intentionally self-inflicted harm without a fatal outcome.

Suicide
Epidemiology
Internationally, suicide rates vary widely, with the highest incidences found in Russia, Lithuania, Belarus, Kazakhstan, Ukraine and Hungary. There are about 5000 suicides a year in England and Wales, an annual incidence of approximately 1/10000 (1% of all deaths). The rate has been falling since 1998. Suicides worldwide are more common in men than women; in the UK rates are about three times higher in men. Suicide

rates in young men have recently risen sharply in most developed countries; the highest rates are nonetheless found in older (aged 65+) men.

Aetiology
Factors implicated in the aetiology of suicide can be classified as social, biological and psychiatric. Emile Durkheim's social model described two main types of suicide: anomic and egoistic.

Anomic suicide reflects a society's disintegration and loss of common values. This is demonstrated by positive correlations between suicide rates and unemployment and homicide rates, by reductions in suicide in wartime (social unity in adversity) and by the higher suicide rates in urban compared to rural communities. The relationship between suicide and unemployment is also found at the individual level, with job loss in men associated with increased suicide risk in them and their partners.

 Psychiatry at a Glance, 4e. By C. Katona, C. Cooper and M. Robertson. Published 2008 Blackwell Publishing. ISBN: 978-1-4501-8117-4

Some of this association is explained by the increased risk of unemployment in the mentally ill.

Egoistic suicide involves individuals' separation from otherwise cohesive social groups and finds some reflection in the higher suicide rates following bereavement and moving house, in immigrants and people living alone, and the divorced or single, compared to people who are married. However, social isolation is also frequently the consequence of major mental illnesses (mood disorders, schizophrenia and substance use disorders).

Altruistic suicide is in undertaken for the good of society (e.g. Kamakazi pilots in the Second World War).

Availability of means will also affect suicide rates: high rates in the USA have been linked to the ease of obtaining firearms; UK recent public health measures have included reduction in the size of paracetamol and aspirin packs. A positive family history of suicide is associated with an increased suicide risk. A large proportion of people who commit suicide have consulted their general practitioners (GPs) in the weeks prior, highlighting the need to recognize people at risk and consequent prevention. Although no consistent biological correlate of suicide has been found, evidence both from brain and cerebrospinal fluid (CSF) studies in suicides and suicide attempters (particularly those using violent means) suggests that serotonergic underactivity (as reflected in levels of 5HT and its metabolites, as well as in 5HT receptors and uptake sites) may be involved.

Assessment

Perhaps the strongest association with suicide is psychiatric illness, with rates increased 50-fold in psychiatric inpatients. Retrospective 'psychiatric autopsy' studies have suggested that a current psychiatric diagnosis can be made in almost all suicides. Specific diagnoses implicated include major depression (with a lifetime suicide risk of 15%), schizophrenia (10%), alcoholism (3–4%) and (less consistently) personality disorder (present in 30–60% of completed suicides), anorexia nervosa and substance misuse. The relationship between depression and suicide is strongest in old age. In contrast, the recent increase in suicide rates in young men is associated with personality disorders and substance misuse. Suicide rates are also increased in people with chronic painful illnesses.

The acronym SAD PERSONS is an *aide-mémoire* for risk factors in suicides: Sex, Age, Depression, Previous attempts, Ethanol abuse, Rational thinking loss (particularly psychosis), Social support lacking, Organized plan, No pastimes and Sickness (with special attention to medical disorders that have been shown to increase risk).

Management

Suicide prevention requires action at the population level (tackling unemployment and reducing access to methods of self-harm), as well as improving detection and treatment of psychiatric disorders, and careful assessment of risk. Urgent hospitalization (consider detention under the Mental Health Act), safe care and intensive pharmaco- and psychotherapy of actively suicidal patients are necessary.

DSH
Epidemiology and correlates

DSH is a much (20–30 times) commoner event than completed suicide, with an annual incidence of 2–3/1000 in the UK, where (in contrast to the USA) most cases involve drug overdose rather than physical self-injury. Unlike completed suicide, DSH is more frequent in women, the under 35s, lower social classes and the single or divorced. Like suicide, DSH is associated with psychiatric illness, particularly depression (usually mild) and personality disorder.

In borderline personality disorder, repetitive self harm (commonly superficial wrist cutting) may be carried out to relieve tension rather than due to a wish to die.

Assessment

The immediate priority is medical stabilization. Subsequent psychiatric assessment first involves establishing a rapport (essential if the DSH is to be a springboard to appropriate management) and suspending any pejorative judgements. Relevant interview topics include identification of motive(s), acute and chronic problems and associated coping strategies, and of current psychiatric illness.

DSH is often precipitated by undesirable life-events. In most cases, its motive can be understood in terms of one or more of a desire to *interrupt* a sequence of events seen as both inevitable and undesirable; a need for *attention* or to *communicate* (decoding and transmission of such communications may itself be effective in reducing subsequent risk); and a true *wish to die*. The latter, although probably the single best indicator of high subsequent risk of suicide, is seldom unequivocal or stable. Subjects at high risk have a clinical profile more characteristic of suicide than of DSH. Specific indicators of high risk include leaving a suicide note, making a will, continued determination to die, marked feelings of hopelessness, clear evidence of psychiatric illness (particularly severe depression) and an attempt carefully prepared with precautions taken to prevent discovery and high lethality risk, either objectively or as imagined by the patient. Risk is higher in older, male, unemployed or socially isolated individuals. Risk of repeated non-fatal DSH is highest in subjects of low social class, with antisocial personality disorder, no work and/or a criminal record, and in those who abuse substances.

Options for management

The objectives of DSH management are to decrease short-term risk of repetition and of completed suicide, to initiate or continue treatment of any underlying psychiatric illness (consider safety in overdose when prescribing antidepressants) and to address ongoing social difficulties. A good first step is to ascertain and then agree with the patient what their problems are and what immediate interventions are both feasible and acceptable to them. Such a 'contract' can include a promise not to repeat any DSH. Ensure that they know whom they can turn to (e.g. A&E) if they fear they may harm themselves again or have already done so. Only a small minority (usually where social support is lacking) need inpatient admission, although where suicide risk is high, compulsory admission may be indicated where the patient has active suicidal plans and intent. Crisis team referral may be needed if suicidal thoughts persist. Brief psychotherapy may be helpful, as may referral to Social Services and/or voluntary agencies (e.g. the Samaritans). The frequency of repetitive DSH in the context of personality disorder may be reduced by simple cognitive (problem-solving) techniques and intensive follow-up. Dialectical behaviour therapy (Chapter 33) can reduce repetitive self-harm in emotionally unstable personality disorder.

Outcome

About 20% of people who have self-harmed repeat their act within one year. Risk of actual suicide within a year is 1–2%, a 100-fold increase compared with the general population. Prior suicide attempt(s) (particularly in the presence of untreated major depressive episode) is the best single predictor of future completed suicide.

6 Schizophrenia: phenomenology and aetiology

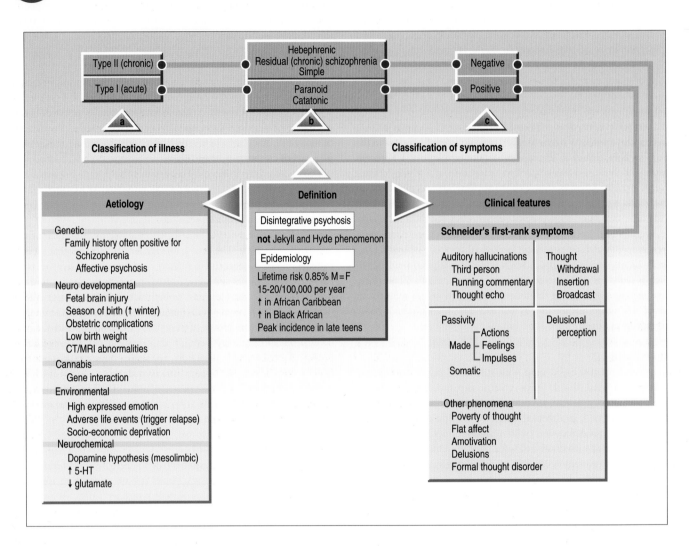

The term psychosis describes the misperception of thoughts and perceptions that arise from the patient's mind/imagination as reality, and includes delusions and hallucinations. About 3% of the general population has clinically significant psychosis; the most common diagnoses are bipolar affective disorder (Chapter 9) and schizophrenia. Others include schizoaffective disorder (affective and schizophrenic symptoms occur together and with equal prominence), delusional disorder (a delusion or delusional system with other areas of thinking and functioning well preserved), brief psychotic episodes (lasting less than the duration required for schizophrenia or other psychotic diagnoses) and drug-induced psychoses (Chapter 17). This chapter concerns schizophrenia.

History and epidemiology

Many lay people misconceive schizophrenia as a 'split personality' in which the individual can behave quite normally but then suddenly becomes bizarre or dangerous. In fact, schizophrenia (literally 'split mind') is characterized by the 'splitting' of normal links between perception, mood, thinking, behaviour and contact with reality. Emil Kraepelin (1893) suggested the distinction between bipolar affective disorder

(manic – depressive illness), where normal function was regained between periods of relapse, and dementia praecox, characterized by the irreversible deterioration of mental functions. The latter corresponds broadly to current concepts of schizophrenia.

Schizophrenia occurs in 15–20/100 000 individuals per year, with a lifetime morbidity risk of 0.85% (male/female) and a peak incidence in late teens or early adulthood.

Clinical features

Kurt Schneider (1959) described the *first-rank symptoms of schizophrenia* (FRS). They include specific types of *auditory hallucination* (a person discussing or making a running commentary about the patient); *thought echo* (hearing one's own thoughts out loud [*echo de la pensée*]); *thought withdrawal, insertion and broadcast* (experiencing thoughts being inserted or removed from one's brain, or believing that one's thoughts are available to others); *passivity* (see Chapter 2); *somatic passivity* (a belief that the patient's body is under the control of others [e.g. others can generate sensations of heat or pain]) and *delusional perception* (ascribing a delusional meaning to a real perception [e.g. 'When I saw a bunch of flowers by the side of the road, I knew the terrorists were after me']). In fact, 8% of patients with non-schizophrenic functional psychoses have one or more FRS, and 20% of people with chronic schizophrenia never show them.

Second-rank symptoms, which are less diagnostically specific, include catatonic behaviour, secondary delusions and other hallucinations.

Formal thought disorder (e.g. loosening of associations [Chapter 2]), neologisms (new words, or ordinary words used in a special way), concrete thinking (inability to deal with abstract ideas) and 'word salad' (jumbled nonsense) can also occur.

Delusions (Chapter 2) in schizophrenia are usually systematized and often bizarre. Content is frequently persecutory (an individual or group intends to harm them [e.g. by poisoning]) or of reference (e.g. patient is mentioned on the television or knows that people are talking about him or her). It is important to distinguish between the term 'paranoid', which refers to self-referential (i.e. persecutory or grandiose) beliefs and persecutory. Other types of delusion may also occur in schizophrenia.

Symptoms can be divided into *positive* (hallucinations, delusions); *negative* (poverty of speech, flat affect, poor motivation, social withdrawal, lack of concern for social conventions); and *cognitive* (poor attention and memory). Significant social and occupational problems are usually present.

Classification

Current diagnostic criteria are still broadly based on Schneider's FRS. ICD-10 requires that a FRS, or a persistent delusion, is present for at least a month. Two 'second-rank symptoms' may also be diagnostic. The diagnosis should not be made in the presence of drug intoxication or withdrawal, overt brain disease or prominent affective symptoms. The DSM-IV criteria are very similar, but require that symptoms are present for at least six months.

Subtypes of schizophrenia include the following:

Paranoid schizophrenia: the most common subtype, in which delusions and auditory hallucinations are evident.

Catatonic schizophrenia: much rarer. Psychomotor disturbances are prominent, often alternating between motor immobility (e.g. stupor) and excessive activity (excitement). Rigidity, posturing (e.g. waxy flexibility – maintaining strange postures), echolalia (copying speech) and echopraxia (copying behaviours) may occur.

Hebephrenic (disorganized) schizophrenia: early onset and poor prognosis. Behaviour is irresponsible and unpredictable; mood inappropriate and affect incongruous, perhaps with giggling, mannerisms and pranks; thought incoherence and fleeting delusions and hallucinations occur.

Residual (chronic) schizophrenia: there is a history of one or more episodes meeting criteria for one of the types of schizophrenia described above, but in the current illness 'negative' and often cognitive symptoms predominate.

Undifferentiated (simple) (deterioration, defect state): uncommon; negative symptoms develop without preceding overt psychotic symptoms.

An alternative classification system has been suggested: *type I* (acute onset, positive symptoms [hallucinations, delusions], normal brain ventricular size, good prognosis and response to neuroleptics, dopamine abnormalities); and *type II* (chronic, negative symptoms, enlarged ventricles, poor prognosis and response to neuroleptics, neurone loss).

Aetiology

There is good evidence for a *genetic component*, with an increased rate of schizophrenia and affective psychoses in relatives of people with schizophrenia. The risk of developing schizophrenia has been estimated as 50% in someone who has a monozygotic twin with the disorder, and 15% if a dizygotic twin is affected. Adoptive studies show that adopted-away offspring of schizophrenics have an increased (about 12%) chance of developing schizophrenia. It is likely that a number of genes affecting brain development contribute to this increased susceptibility.

Neurodevelopmental hypothesis

Factors that interfere with early brain development lead to abnormalities which are expressed in the mature brain. Evidence for this includes increased rates of schizophrenia in those born in the winter and hence more likely to be exposed to maternal influenza during mid-pregnancy, or with obstetric complications, low birthweight and perinatal injuries. Developmental delay, poor academic performance, 'soft' neurological signs (e.g. abnormal movements, mixed-handedness) and temporal lobe epilepsy are associated with schizophrenia. The neurodevelopmental hypothesis is also supported by findings of increased ventricular size and small amounts of grey matter loss from CT/MRI studies.

People who smoke cannabis in adolescence are more likely to develop schizophrenia, probably because cannabis interferes with neurodevelopment. People who are homozygous for a variant of the COMT (catechol-O-methyl transferase) gene are ten times more likely to develop schizophrenia if they smoke cannabis. This is an example of an environment/gene interaction.

Social factors

Schizophrenia is also associated with socio-economic deprivation and an excess of life-events in the three weeks before the onset of acute symptoms. In the UK, the incidence of all psychoses is significantly higher in African-Caribbean and Black African populations compared with the White population (see Chapter 23). People with schizophrenia living in families with high expressed emotion (EE, relatives over-involved or making hostile or excessive critical comments) are more likely to relapse.

The way in which genetic, neurodevelopmental and social factors result in schizophrenia in vulnerable individuals is not clearly understood, but the final common pathway appears to involve dopamine excess or over-activity in the mesolimbic pathways (stimulant drugs such as amphetamines release dopamine and lead to psychosis; antipsychotics, which block dopamine receptors, treat psychosis successfully; increased dopamine receptors have been found at post-mortem. Raised 5HT and decreased glutamate activity have also been implicated.

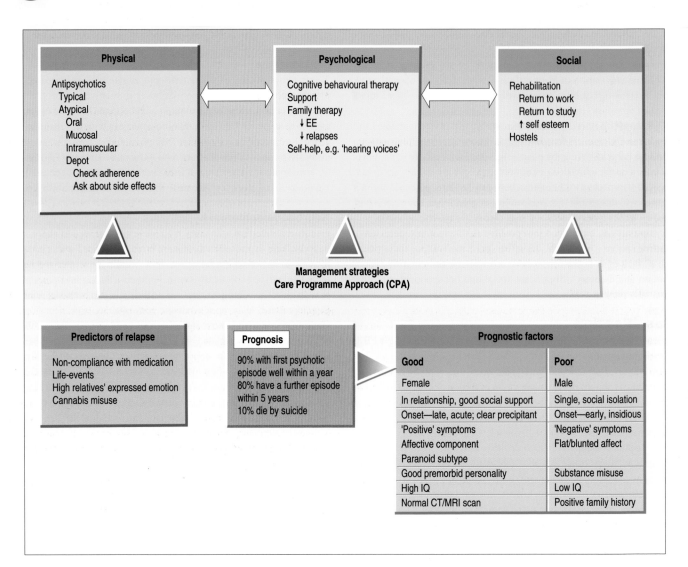

Physical

Antipsychotics
  Typical
  Atypical
    Oral
    Mucosal
    Intramuscular
    Depot
      Check adherence
      Ask about side effects

Psychological

Cognitive behavioural therapy
Support
Family therapy
  ↓ EE
  ↓ relapses
Self-help, e.g. 'hearing voices'

Social

Rehabilitation
  Return to work
  Return to study
  ↑ self esteem
Hostels

Management strategies
Care Programme Approach (CPA)

Predictors of relapse

Non-compliance with medication
Life-events
High relatives' expressed emotion
Cannabis misuse

Prognosis

90% with first psychotic
episode well within a year
80% have a further episode
within 5 years
10% die by suicide

Prognostic factors

Good	Poor
Female	Male
In relationship, good social support	Single, social isolation
Onset—late, acute; clear precipitant	Onset—early, insidious
'Positive' symptoms	'Negative' symptoms
Affective component	Flat/blunted affect
Paranoid subtype	
Good premorbid personality	Substance misuse
High IQ	Low IQ
Normal CT/MRI scan	Positive family history

Management

Management requires *antipsychotic medication* (see Chapter 34) and *psychological and social interventions*.

Medication

Antipsychotics are the mainstay of treatment. They are effective in treating 'positive symptoms' in the acute episode (e.g. hallucinations, delusions, passivity phenomena) and in preventing relapses. Typical (conventional) and atypical (second-generation) antipsychotics (see Chapter 34) are equally effective in the treatment of positive symptoms, but have different side-effect profiles. 'Atypical' antipsychotics cause fewer motor side-effects, but some are associated with weight gain and diabetes. Only clozapine, the prototypical atypical antipsychotic drug, has been shown to be effective in the treatment of psychosis that does not respond to treatment with other antipsychotic drugs. Atypical antipsychotics may be effective in the treatment of negative symptoms, although evidence for this is equivocal for drugs other than clozapine. Patients who are agitated, overactive or violent may require sedation (with typical or atypical antipsychotics or with benzodiazepines). (Note: the patient receiving clozapine requires supervised haematological monitoring [see Chapter 34].)

Medication may be administered *orally*, *intramuscularly* or by long-acting *depot injections* (see Chapter 34). Depot preparations provide long-term prophylaxis, increase adherence, allow regular contact with either community psychiatric nurses (CPNs) or clinics and avoid first pass metabolism. However, most patients prefer oral medication. Treatment should be commenced as soon as possible after diagnosis as there is evidence that long periods between symptom onset and effective treatment are associated with worse outcomes. Treatment is with the lowest dose that effectively controls symptoms to minimize side-effects, as these are associated with poor treatment adherence. If the patient experiences extrapyramidal side-effects (e.g. dystonia, oculogyric crisis), anticholinergic drugs (e.g. procyclidine, benztropine) should be given immediately, intramuscularly if necessary. Regular antiparkinsonian drugs should be avoided as they cause unwanted side-effects (e.g. blurred vision, dry mouth), may be abused and may worsen or provoke tardive dyskinesia (TD). TD may respond to the reduction/cessation of antipsychotics or to tetrabenazine, but is irreversible in up to 50% of cases. As weight gain, cardiac arrythmias and diabetes may also be problematic during treatment with atypical antipsychotic drugs, patients require regular monitoring of weight, lipid and glucose profiles and ECGs. People with schizophrenia can become depressed and may require antidepressant medication. Rarely, *electroconvulsive therapy* (ECT) may be useful (e.g. in catatonic stupor, excitement).

Psychological treatment

Cognitive behavioural therapy (CBT) is often useful in helping patients cope with persistent delusions and hallucinations. The aim is to alleviate distress and disability, and not necessarily to eliminate symptoms. Psychological support is important for all people with schizophrenia and their families. Family therapy helps the family reduce their excessive expressed emotion (EE), and there is good evidence that it is effective in preventing relapses. Self-help (e.g. Hearing Voices groups) can be helpful for people with psychosis to share experiences and ways to cope with symptoms. Psychoanalysis is rarely useful.

Social support

Helping people to return to work or study is crucial in maintaining their self-esteem and quality of life. Where this is not possible, day centres can provide daytime structure.

Appropriate accommodation is important. People with residual symptoms (e.g. negative or cognitive symptoms) may not be able to live independently. Inpatient and community rehabilitation services aim to maximize independence (e.g. by teaching daily living skills). A range of supported living arrangements, from 24-hour staffed hostels to independent housing with support workers who visit once a week, are available depending on need.

People with psychosis are treated in the community rather than in hospital wherever possible, although admission may be necessary if the risks of serious neglect, suicide/DSH or harm to others are high. If the patient refuses treatment, formal admission under the Mental Health Act may be required. Delivering a positive and non-stigmatizing treatment experience is critical for the patient's subsequent engagement with the treating team and adherence to treatment. All patients receiving secondary psychiatric services are managed through the Care Programme Approach (CPA) system. This means that they are assigned a care coordinator who will visit them, provide support, monitor their mental state and treatment adherence, and help with practical aspects of daily life (see Chapter 38).

Prognosis

Ninety per cent of people experiencing a first psychotic episode will be well within a year, but about 80% have a further episode within five years. Recent studies suggest that 75% of patients will discontinue their initial medication within the first 18 months, and those who discontinue antipsychotic medication altogether may be five times more likely to relapse over this period. In addition to taking medication, avoiding illicit drug use (in particular cannabis) and excessive stress will reduce the risk of relapse.

Cohort studies investigating outcomes more than ten years after diagnosis with schizophrenia have found that a minority (about 15%) of patients recover completely, about 50% have continued episodes of relapse with no or relatively minor disability between relapses; and 25% have a chronic illness with persistent symptoms and significant disability. Better prognosis is encountered in the developing world; this may be due to social structure, family support and/or less stigma. Good prognostic factors include an acute onset, 'positive' symptoms, a strong affective component (e.g. depressed), paranoid subtype, good premorbid personality, birth trauma, higher intelligence and a normal MRI/CT scan.

Poor prognostic factors include male gender, younger age at onset, being single, social isolation, illicit drug use, an insidious early onset without precipitants, negative symptoms, low socio-economic class, abnormal premorbid personality and a positive family history of schizophrenia.

The lifetime suicide risk is 10%. Suicide risk is higher in young men with persistent hallucinations or delusions and in those with a history of illicit drug use and previous suicide attempts, especially just before/during the first three months after discharge.

8 Depression

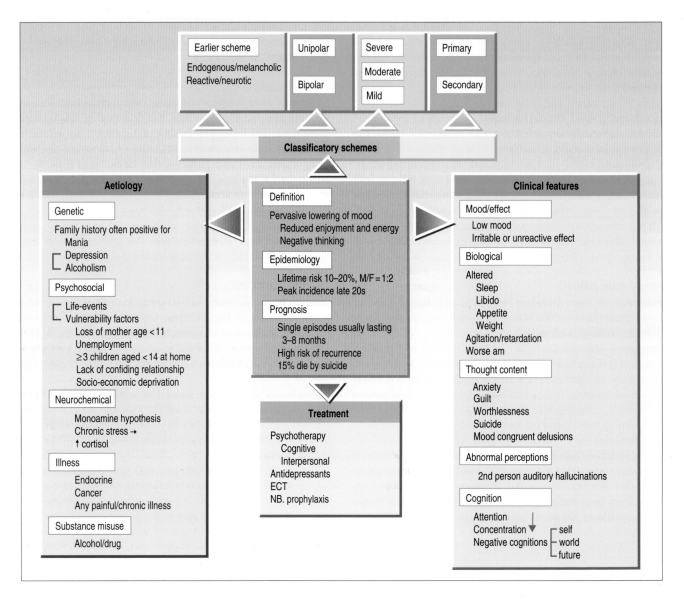

Definitions and classification

The most common symptom of depression is a pervasive lowering of mood, although in modern classification systems this is not essential for a diagnosis to be made. ICD-10 classifies depressive disorders according to severity, and identifies three core symptoms: low mood, anhedonia (loss of enjoyment in formerly pleasurable activities) and decreased energy (or increased fatiguability). A diagnosis of mild depressive episode requires two of the three core symptoms and two from the following list: reduced concentration and attention; reduced self-esteem and self-confidence; ideas of guilt and worthlessness; feelings of hopelessness regarding the future; thoughts of self-harm, disrupted sleep and increased or decreased appetite. For a moderate depressive episode, six symptoms, including at least two of the core symptoms, should be present, which together should cause considerable interference with usual activities. A severe depressive episode specifies at least eight symptoms, including all three core symptoms, causing marked distress or interference with daily activities. Depression associated with psy-

chotic features is always classified as severe. Each grade of severity requires symptoms to be present every day for at least two weeks. The DSM-IV-TR classification system is similar.

Mood disorders with recurrent episodes are described as unipolar if they include only depressive episodes, or bipolar if there is a history of at least one manic or hypomanic episode. Earlier classification systems proposed a distinction between 'endogenous' and 'neurotic/reactive' depression. The former is more severe, less likely to have external precipitants and is characterized by prominent, 'biological' features (see below), whereas the latter is milder, more understandable in terms of external circumstances and may show symptomatic overlap with anxiety.

Clinical features

Although depressed mood, anhedonia and increased fatiguability are regarded as the hallmarks of depression, these symptoms, can be masked by severe anxiety, excess consumption of alcohol, hypochondriacal preoccupations or irritability. Anhedonia is usually accompanied by loss of motivation and emotional reactivity. Biological symptoms involve sleep, appetite and libido, and may be particularly prominent in the elderly, who less often complain of disturbed mood. Sleep is classically decreased, with a pattern of early waking (more than two hours before usual) and maximal lowering of mood in the morning (diurnal variation). Appetite is reduced and often associated with weight loss; in severe cases, there is reluctance or even refusal to eat or drink. Libido is reduced or absent. Motor activity is often altered, with psychomotor agitation or retardation (of speech and/or movement), or both. The pattern may be reversed with initial anxiety-related insomnia, subsequent oversleeping, increased appetite and a relatively bright and reactive mood. DSM-IV-TR calls this atypical depression and ICD-10 suggests that it is particularly common in adolescence.

Thought content often includes negative, pessimistic thoughts about the self (low self-esteem), the world and the future (Beck's cognitive triad), guilt and worthlessness or death or suicide. Cognition may be impaired, with reduced attention, concentration and decisiveness. Psychotic features may occur and are usually mood-congruent. Delusions are usually nihilistic (e.g. a belief that the patient is dead, has lost all their assets or their body is rotting) or hypochondriacal, concerning illness or death. Where hallucinations occur they are usually auditory, in the second person and accusing, condemning or urging suicide (e.g. 'You are bad, you might as well be dead').

Differential diagnosis

Several organic conditions may present with depressive symptoms and are considered briefly below. Depression may be difficult to distinguish from normal sadness, particularly in the context of bereavement (Chapter 10) or severe physical illness. The diagnosis depends on finding a pattern of characteristic features and on the degree and duration of associated disability. Predominant negative, guilty or suicidal thoughts favour a diagnosis of depression, but such symptoms may be difficult to elicit if depression is severe. Similarly, depressive retardation may be difficult to distinguish from the flat (unreactive) affect sometimes found in chronic schizophrenia (Chapter 6). Alcohol or drug withdrawal may mimic depression, but substance use (especially alcohol and/or sedatives) is highly comorbid with depression. Depression is often also comorbid with panic disorder, agoraphobia, obsessive compulsive disorder (OCD), eating disorders and personality disorders.

Epidemiology

The lifetime risk of depression is about 10–20%, with rates almost doubled in women. First onset is typically in the third decade (earlier for bipolar disorder), with point prevalence higher in middle and old age. Depression is commoner in urban than in rural areas, and particularly in women from lower socio-economic classes.

Aetiology

A genetic contribution is evident in both twin and adoption studies, but less markedly for unipolar than bipolar depression. Neurochemical and neuroendocrine mechanisms have been proposed. The dominant neurochemical theory is the 'monoamine hypothesis' based on the observations (made in the 1960s) that monoamine (particularly noradrenalin and serotonin) metabolites in cerebrospinal fluid (CSF) and urine are reduced in depressed patients, and that antidepressants increase monoamine availability. This has been modified to emphasize changes to monoamine neuroreceptors (particularly β-adrenoreceptors and $5HT_2$ receptors) that occur in depression and normalize with antidepressant treatment. Chronic stress leads to increased cortisol levels, and these may cause depressed mood through decreased expression of neurotrophins, which are important in neuronal growth. Antidepressants increase monoamine availability and this may lead to improved mood through increased expression of neurotrophins. Neuroendocrine abnormalities found in some depressed patients include hypercortisolaemia and impaired thyroid axis activity. Depression is also associated with characteristic sleep-electroencephalographic (EEG) changes and reduced frontal lobe blood flow; however, to date there are no reliable diagnostic biomarkers of depression.

The most important psychosocial factors implicated are recent adverse life events (e.g. bereavement or deteriorating physical health), parental loss and major stress or abuse in childhood (which appears to increase vulnerability to depression in response to life-events). Adverse current social circumstances, especially unemployment and lack of a confiding relationship, increase vulnerability. Several physical illnesses (most endocrine disorders, many cancers, some viral infections) and some medications (including steroids, some antihypertensives and the oral contraceptive) are specifically associated with depression. Women are particularly vulnerable to episodes of depression in the weeks following childbirth.

Management

Most depressive illnesses can be managed in primary care, although many are undetected. Detection rates can be enhanced by remembering that depressed patients often present with other conditions, or through screening questionnaires. Management starts with risk assessment in terms of self-neglect and, most importantly, suicide. Psychiatric referral is indicated if suicide risk is high or if the depression is severe, unresponsive to initial treatment or recurrent. Comorbid physical illnesses or substance misuse problems should be addressed. Selective serotonin reuptake inhibitors (SSRIs) are now the most commonly prescribed drugs for depression (see Chapter 35) and can have a 60–70% response rate, but frequently fail because of inadequate dosage, duration or adherence. Electroconvulsive therapy (ECT) is very effective in severe cases, particularly where psychosis or stupor is present, and can be life-saving if fluids and food are being refused. Refractory depression may also respond to combination treatments such as lithium augmentation.

Specific psychological techniques (including cognitive behavioural therapy [CBT], interpersonal and problem-solving psychotherapy) have similar success rates to antidepressants in non-psychotic depression, and are recommended in preference to antidepressants as a first-line treatment for mild depression, and in conjunction with antidepressants in more serious illness. CBT also has some prophylactic effect.

Continuing antidepressants for at least six months after a first episode reduces the relapse rate; in recurrent depression prophylactic effects have been demonstrated for up to five years. When discontinuing antidepressants, taper slowly to avoid withdrawal symptoms.

Prognosis

Single episodes of depression usually last 3–8 months. About 20% of patients remain depressed for two years or more and about 50% have recurrences; this rises to 80% in severe cases, such as in those requiring inpatient care. Recurrent episodes tend to become increasingly severe with shortening of disease-free periods, emphasizing the importance of prophylactic treatment. Lifetime suicide risk is 15% in severe depression, but much lower in milder illness. Successful acute and long-term treatment of depression reduces suicide and overall morbidity and mortality. Predictors of poor outcome include early onset, initial symptom severity and psychiatric or physical comorbidity.

9 Bipolar affective disorder

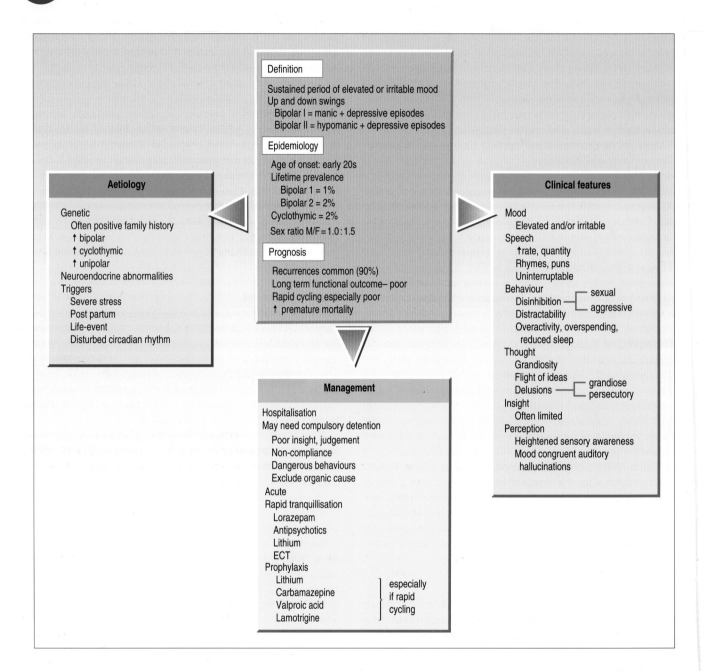

Definition

Sustained period of elevated or irritable mood
Up and down swings
  Bipolar I = manic + depressive episodes
  Bipolar II = hypomanic + depressive episodes

Epidemiology

Age of onset: early 20s
Lifetime prevalence
  Bipolar 1 = 1%
  Bipolar 2 = 2%
Cyclothymic = 2%
Sex ratio M/F = 1.0 : 1.5

Prognosis

Recurrences common (90%)
Long term functional outcome– poor
Rapid cycling especially poor
↑ premature mortality

Aetiology

Genetic
  Often positive family history
    ↑ bipolar
    ↑ cyclothymic
    ↑ unipolar
Neuroendocrine abnormalities
Triggers
  Severe stress
  Post partum
  Life-event
  Disturbed circadian rhythm

Clinical features

Mood
  Elevated and/or irritable
Speech
  ↑rate, quantity
  Rhymes, puns
  Uninterruptable
Behaviour
  Disinhibition ── sexual / aggressive
  Distractability
  Overactivity, overspending,
    reduced sleep
Thought
  Grandiosity
  Flight of ideas
  Delusions ── grandiose / persecutory
Insight
  Often limited
Perception
  Heightened sensory awareness
  Mood congruent auditory
    hallucinations

Management

Hospitalisation
May need compulsory detention
  Poor insight, judgement
  Non-compliance
  Dangerous behaviours
  Exclude organic cause
Acute
Rapid tranquillisation
  Lorazepam
  Antipsychotics
  Lithium
  ECT
Prophylaxis
  Lithium
  Carbamazepine   } especially
  Valproic acid   if rapid
  Lamotrigine   cycling

Definitions and classification

The bipolar affective disorders are characterized by recurrent episodes of altered mood and activity, involving both upswings and downswings. Recent classificatory systems (ICD-10, DSM-IV) have therefore had to define both individual episodes and patterns of recurrence.

Individual episodes are classified as *major depressive* (see Chapter 8), *manic*, hypomanic (less severe) or (more rarely) *mixed*, where features of both mania and major depression are present or alternate rapidly. In ICD-10, bipolar affective disorder is defined as at least two episodes, including at least one hypomanic or manic episode. In DSM-IV-TR patterns of recurrence can be classified as *bipolar I* disorder (with one or more manic or mixed episodes and usually one or more major depressive episodes); *bipolar II* disorder (recurrent major depressive and hypomanic but not manic episodes); and *cyclothymic* disorder, with chronic mood fluctuations over at least two years, unrelated to external circumstances, including individual episodes of depression and hypomania (but not mania) of insufficient severity to meet diagnostic criteria.

Clinical features

The cardinal clinical feature of a manic episode is alteration in mood, which is usually elated and expansive, but may also be characterized by intense irritability. Associated features include increased psychomotor activity (rapid thinking and speech, distractibility, decreased need for sleep); exaggerated optimism, inflated self-esteem and decreased social inhibition, with apparent disregard for potentially harmful conse-

 Psychiatry at a Glance, 4e. By C. Katona, C. Cooper and M. Robertson. Published 2008 Blackwell Publishing. ISBN: 978-1-4501-8117-4

quences (sexual over-activity, reckless spending, dangerous driving and/or inappropriate business, religious or political initiatives). Mood-congruent or incongruent psychotic features (including Schneiderian first-rank symptoms [see Chapter 6]) may also be found and, if present with equal prominence, suggest a diagnosis of schizoaffective disorder.

Heightened sensory awareness is common. Speech abnormalities include uninterruptibility (pressure) and flight of ideas (jumping from topic to topic [see Chapter 2]). Insight is often absent. Manic and hypomanic episodes are distinguished on the basis that mania is more severe, causing marked disruption to work and social or interpersonal life, with possible psychotic features and consequently usually requires hospitalization; hypomania is less severe and disruptive and psychotic symptoms are absent. The depressive episode (phase) of bipolar I disorder is usually associated with psychomotor retardation, while agitation is more commonly seen in bipolar II depression. In 20% of cases (mostly mood-congruent) psychotic symptoms are also present (e.g. auditory hallucination, ['You are a star. Why don't you fly?']).

Differential diagnosis

It is important to exclude substance abuse (particularly amphetamines or cocaine) and mood abnormalities secondary to endocrine disturbance (idiopathic Cushing's syndrome or steroid-induced psychoses) or epilepsy. 'Secondary' mania or organic mood disorder may be precipitated by severe physical illness, particularly stroke. Acute schizophrenia may present very much like mania: persecutory or grandiose delusions, auditory hallucinations and increased psychomotor activity may occur in both conditions. Schizoaffective disorder should be diagnosed where affective and schizophreniform symptoms are equally prominent. Personality disorders (emotionally unstable or histrionic) may mimic some features of the mood or behavioural disturbance of mania and hypomania. Other disorders to consider include attention-deficit hyperactivity disorder (ADHD) in younger people and transient psychoses induced by extreme stress, although in both elevation of mood is rare. Bipolar disorder can be also comorbid with conditions including substance use, personality disorders, obsessive compulsive disorder and anxiety.

Epidemiology

The lifetime prevalence of bipolar I disorder is about 1%, with a further 2% experiencing bipolar II disorder and 2% cyclothymia in their lifetime. The female:male ratio is about 1.5:1.0, the female excess being more prominent in the bipolar II group. Peak age of onset is in the early twenties. Several studies have shown greater prevalence rates in higher social classes, probably reflecting differences in access to diagnosis.

Aetiology

There is clear evidence of a strong familial component. Rates of both bipolar disorder (including cyclothymia) and unipolar depression are commoner than expected in first-degree relatives of bipolar subjects. Both sex-linked and autosomal inheritance have been proposed. A number of neuroendocrine abnormalities have been described, including hypercortisolaemia, increased aldosterone secretion and blunted growth hormone response to hypoglycaemia. The findings are less consistent than in depressive illness.

Some studies suggest that manic episodes may be precipitated by severe stress. In particular, there is a markedly increased risk of manic episodes in the early postpartum weeks; this may relate to dopamine receptor super-sensitivity associated with postpartum falls in oestrogen and progesterone levels (Chapter 25). There appears to be an increase in manic episodes in the spring and early summer. Disturbance of circadian rhythms (e.g. in jet lag and sleep loss) may precipitate an episode, as may a recent life-event. Psychodynamic models of mania suggest denial of loss or loss-associated conflict in order to avoid depression, or loss of superego ('conscience') control. Psychogenic models of mania are not frequently invoked in mainstream psychiatry.

Management

Acute mania usually requires hospitalization, although the introduction of crisis and home treatment teams has enabled some people to be treated at home. Since patients often lose insight early, detention without consent may be required under the Mental Health Act. Exclusion of organic causes is vital. Antipsychotics (typical or atypical, in similar doses to those used in schizophrenia) form the mainstay of acute management of both mania and hypomania. Antipsychotics are effective in controlling overactivity and agitation and (somewhat more slowly) in reducing elation and disinhibition. Lorazepam and antipsychotics may be useful for rapid tranquillization (see Chapter 34).

Lithium is effective as an acute antimanic agent, although it lacks the potential for very rapid behavioural control. Maintenance treatment with lithium has been shown in many controlled trials to reduce the frequency and severity of subsequent episodes. Its 'real-life' effectiveness is more difficult to demonstrate and probably depends on careful supervision and education for good adherence. Lithium therapy (which may also be useful in cyclothymia) requires comprehensive pre-initiation screening (including renal and thyroid function estimation) and regular monitoring in view of both of its narrow therapeutic range and its long-term potential to induce hypothyroidism.

A number of anticonvulsants (carbamazepine, sodium valproate and lamotrigine) appear to be effective in preventing relapses of mania or depression. Anticonvulsants may also be preferable to lithium where rapid cycling occurs (see below). Episodes of depression in bipolar disorder are treated similarly to unipolar depression, but since antidepressants may precipitate mania or rapid cycling, they are generally given in combination with a mood stabilizer. Psychotherapeutic support is important in helping patients come to terms with their illness and sometimes the embarrassment or remorse associated with past manic behaviour (e.g. indiscretions).

Prognosis

The lifetime prognosis following a single manic episode is poor, with 90% of patients having manic or depressive recurrences (averaging four episodes in ten years). In bipolar I disorder, both frequency and severity of episodes tend to increase for the first four or five episodes, but then plateau. Long-term functional prognosis (work, family, etc.) is almost as poor as in schizophrenia. A minority who develop 'rapid cycling', with four or more episodes a year, have a particularly poor prognosis and seldom respond to lithium. There is an overall increase in premature mortality, only partially explained by a suicide rate of 10%. Successful lithium prophylaxis (reflecting self-selection for good prognosis as well as good response to lithium) not only modifies severity and duration of episodes, but appears to reduce both suicide and overall mortality. Prognosis for bipolar II disorder is better, although there remains a high suicide risk. Cyclothymia runs a chronic course and approximately 30% risk developing full-blown bipolar disorder.

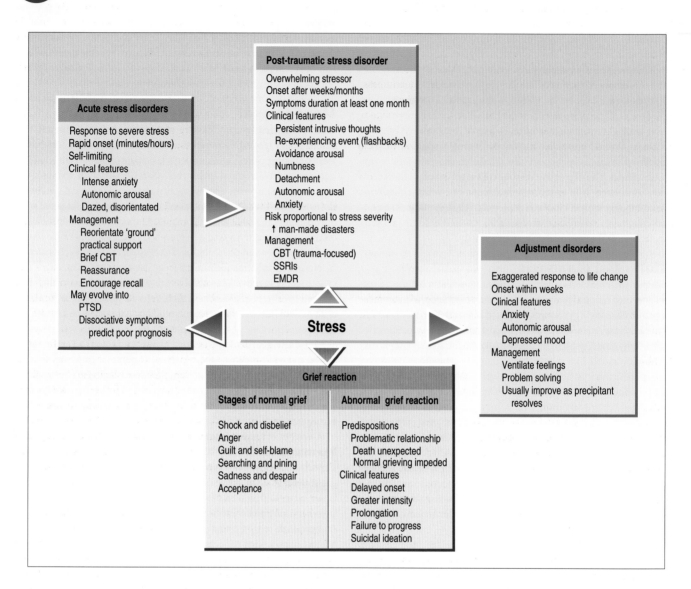

Post-traumatic stress disorder

Overwhelming stressor
Onset after weeks/months
Symptoms duration at least one month
Clinical features
    Persistent intrusive thoughts
    Re-experiencing event (flashbacks)
    Avoidance arousal
    Numbness
    Detachment
    Autonomic arousal
    Anxiety
Risk proportional to stress severity
    ↑ man-made disasters
Management
    CBT (trauma-focused)
    SSRIs
    EMDR

Acute stress disorders

Response to severe stress
Rapid onset (minutes/hours)
Self-limiting
Clinical features
    Intense anxiety
    Autonomic arousal
    Dazed, disorientated
Management
    Reorientate 'ground'
    practical support
    Brief CBT
    Reassurance
    Encourage recall
May evolve into
    PTSD
    Dissociative symptoms
        predict poor prognosis

Adjustment disorders

Exaggerated response to life change
Onset within weeks
Clinical features
    Anxiety
    Autonomic arousal
    Depressed mood
Management
    Ventilate feelings
    Problem solving
    Usually improve as precipitant
        resolves

Stress

Grief reaction

Stages of normal grief	Abnormal grief reaction
Shock and disbelief	Predispositions
Anger	Problematic relationship
Guilt and self-blame	Death unexpected
Searching and pining	Normal grieving impeded
Sadness and despair	Clinical features
Acceptance	Delayed onset
	Greater intensity
	Prolongation
	Failure to progress
	Suicidal ideation

Major psychological stress involves threat or loss. Reactions to a broad range of major stressors (physical or sexual assault, transport accidents, natural disasters, war) are often similar in nature and involve emotional responses (fear from threat and sadness at loss), physical symptoms (autonomic arousal and/or fatigue) and psychological responses, which may be conscious (e.g. avoidance behaviour) or unconscious (e.g. denial or dissociation). Abnormal stress reactions represent exaggerated or maladaptive responses. They may be acute and self-limiting (acute stress reactions) or prolonged (post-traumatic stress disorder [PTSD], adjustment disorder or abnormal grief).

Acute stress reactions

ICD-10 criteria for acute stress reactions require rapid onset (within minutes or hours) of extreme responses to sudden and severe stressful events. There is a mixed and usually changing picture; in addition to the initial state of dazedness, depression, anxiety, anger, despair, over-activity and withdrawal may all be seen, but no one type of symptom

predominates for long. Intense subjective anxiety is accompanied by autonomic arousal (sweating, dry mouth, tachycardia, vomiting). Dissociative symptoms, which predict increased risk of PTSD, include feeling dazed and perplexed, and wandering aimlessly. Purposeless over-activity, reduced sleep and nightmares are also common. Initial management involves helping to reorient and 'ground' the individual. Practical support may be required in dealing with underlying difficulties (e.g. temporary housing following a natural disaster). There is no evidence that anxiolytics or hypnotics are effective and they carry a risk of dependence. In most cases symptoms resolve rapidly (within a few hours at the most) in those cases where removal from the stressful environment is possible; in cases where the stress continues or cannot by its nature be reversed, the symptoms usually begin to diminish after 24–48 hours and are minimal after about three days. Increasing evidence suggests that brief cognitive behaviour therapy (CBT) improves outcome and reduces the rate of chronic PTSD. Persistence of symptoms for more than one month indicates the development of PTSD (see opposite page).

Adjustment disorders

Adjustment disorders include a range of abnormal psychological responses to adversity. They may follow common life changes (e.g. job loss, house move or divorce). The onset is usually within weeks of the stressful event and the duration is usually less than six months, unless there are factors leading to persistence (e.g. ongoing litigation). The presentation includes a broad mix of symptoms of anxiety (autonomic arousal, insomnia, irritability) and depression (sadness, tearfulness, worry). Biological features of depression are usually absent; indeed, the diagnosis should be made only where there are insufficient symptoms to justify a diagnosis of another specific anxiety or depressive disorder. Adjustment disorders usually improve following resolution of their precipitating cause.

Initial management may involve encouragement to ventilate feelings and to develop appropriate coping mechanisms. Such help may focus on 'problem-solving' in which patients are encouraged to form strategies to deal with particular problems. Sometimes formal CBT is required.

Adjustment to chronic or terminal illness may manifest as anxiety, depression or exaggerated disability. There may be a sequence (similar to that in bereavement) of shock and denial (and search for an ever-elusive cure), followed by anger, sadness and acceptance. Management involves adequate symptomatic (particularly pain) control, honest explanation, supportive psychotherapy and family counselling.

PTSD

The onset of PTSD may occur weeks, months or (rarely) years after a severe stressful experience which is of exceptionally threatening or catastrophic nature, and can include assault, accident, disaster, act of terrorism or battle. In DSM-IV-TR, the immediate element of shock is emphasized in the requirement for there to be a subjective experience of intense fear, horror or helplessness. Duration of symptoms for at least one month is required to make the diagnosis. The characteristic features of PTSD involve:

1 *Persistent intrusive thinking or re-experiencing* of the trauma, such as traumatic memories, recurrent dreams or nightmares and re-enactments ('flashbacks') of the traumatic event.

2 *Avoidance* of reminders of the event (e.g. victims not going near the scene of an accident), and thoughts, feelings and conversations associated with the trauma; *numbing, detachment and estrangement* from others, and *loss of interest* in significant activities and sense of a foreshortened future.

3 *Increased arousal* with autonomic symptoms, hyper-vigilance, sleep disturbance, irritability, poor concentration and exaggerated startle response.

There is considerable symptomatic overlap between the avoidance and numbing symptoms of PTSD and depression (see Chapter 8); the latter may also be precipitated by extreme stress and may rather coexist with or be secondary to PTSD.

Risk for PTSD is proportional to the magnitude of the stressor, but may be greater following man-made rather than natural disasters and if some stress continues. Lack of social support and the presence of other adversities at the time of the trauma are crucial vulnerability factors, as is premorbid personality. Many PTSD victims recover over the first few months. If the syndrome persists over 1–2 years, then it may continue in the long term, possibly for the rest of the victim's life, as with many Holocaust survivors. Trauma-focused CBT, eye movement desensitization and reprocessing (EMDR; see Chapter 37) and antidepressant drugs, typically SSRIs (even in the absence of depressive disorder), have been shown to be effective. Debriefing is no longer indicated as it does not, as previously thought, prevent PTSD. (In debriefing, patients were encouraged to recall the stressful events in detail soon after the trauma and supported through the associated emotions.) Alcohol or substance misuse may also be a long-term complication and should be considered.

Bereavement and grief

Bereavement is associated with increased mortality (from cardiovascular disease and cancer) and may precipitate depression and even suicide.

'Normal' grief often follows a recognizable sequence of stages that last for up to two years. The initial reaction to bereavement (lasting days or a few weeks) is of *shock* and *disbelief* with autonomic arousal, but usually without psychological fear. There may be paroxysms of weeping. This may be followed by *anger* at being deserted by the deceased, and *guilt* and *self-blame* for not having done more for them. The next stage consists of '*searching*' or '*pining*', vivid dreams that the dead person is still alive and, often, pseudo-hallucinations (usually at night and always with preserved insight) of seeing or speaking to the dead person. *Sadness* and *despair* follow, accompanied by many features (poor sleep and appetite, social withdrawal) of depression. Finally, *acceptance* occurs that the deceased will not come back, accompanied by a return of interests. Symptoms often recur briefly on anniversaries. The sequence of stages is often less clear-cut than this linear model suggests. Bereavement may be characterized by jumbled feelings as people pass in and out of these stages of grieving.

'Abnormal' grief is characterized by delayed onset, greater intensity of symptoms or prolongation of the reaction. Suicidal ideas may be harboured during abnormal pining (a wish to be with the deceased) or despair. Abnormal grief is more likely where the relationship with the deceased was problematic (ambivalent or over-involved), the death sudden or normal grieving was impeded by social constraints (e.g. 'having to put on a brave face for the children'). In DSM-IV-R and ICD-10, abnormal grief reaction is coded as an adjustment disorder.

Normal grieving requires no specific management apart from support and encouragement to ventilate feelings and accept them as normal. Abnormal grief reactions may respond to CBT, encouraging structured review of the relationship and giving vent to the emotions produced. Antidepressants may be indicated if depressive symptoms are prominent and persistent. Significant suicidal ideation may warrant hospitalization.

11 Anxiety disorders

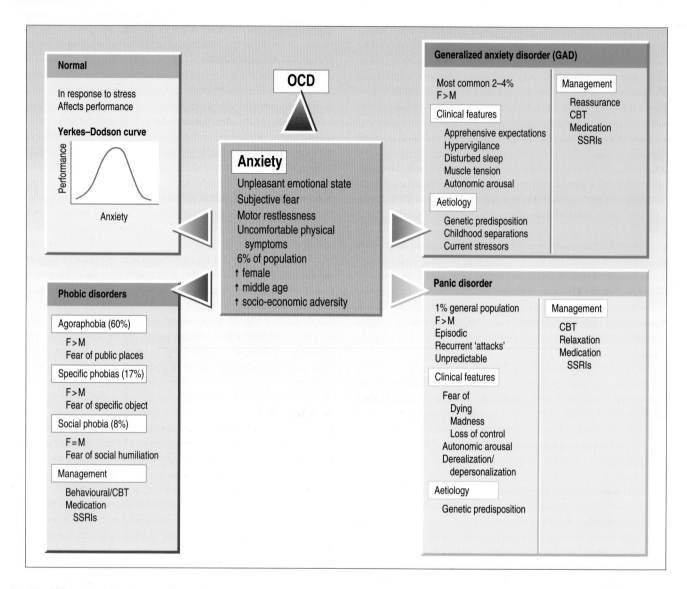

Normal

In response to stress
Affects performance

Yerkes–Dodson curve

Performance / Anxiety

Phobic disorders

Agoraphobia (60%)
   F > M
   Fear of public places

Specific phobias (17%)
   F > M
   Fear of specific object

Social phobia (8%)
   F = M
   Fear of social humiliation

Management
   Behavioural/CBT
   Medication
      SSRIs

OCD

Anxiety
Unpleasant emotional state
Subjective fear
Motor restlessness
Uncomfortable physical
   symptoms
6% of population
↑ female
↑ middle age
↑ socio-economic adversity

Generalized anxiety disorder (GAD)

Most common 2–4%
F > M

Clinical features
   Apprehensive expectations
   Hypervigilance
   Disturbed sleep
   Muscle tension
   Autonomic arousal

Aetiology
   Genetic predisposition
   Childhood separations
   Current stressors

Management
   Reassurance
   CBT
   Medication
      SSRIs

Panic disorder

1% general population
F > M
Episodic
Recurrent 'attacks'
Unpredictable

Clinical features
   Fear of
      Dying
      Madness
      Loss of control
   Autonomic arousal
   Derealization/
      depersonalization

Aetiology
   Genetic predisposition

Management
   CBT
   Relaxation
   Medication
      SSRIs

Definition and classification

Anxiety is an unpleasant emotional state involving subjective fear, bodily discomfort and physical symptoms. There is often a feeling of impending threat or death, which may or may not be in response to a recognizable threat. The Yerkes–Dodson curve of anxiety against performance illustrates that anxiety can be beneficial up to a plateau of optimal function, beyond which, with increasing anxiety, there is a marked deterioration in performance. Pathological anxiety can present in discrete attacks with no external stimulus (panic disorder), in discrete attacks with feared stimuli (phobias) or in a generalized, persistent state (generalized anxiety disorder [GAD]). Anxiety symptoms also occur in other disorders (e.g. depression).

Epidemiology

Around 6% of the general population experience an anxiety disorder. GAD is the commonest, affecting 2–4%. Other anxiety disorders are phobias (agoraphobia, social phobia, specific phobias), panic disorder and obsessive compulsive disorder (OCD) (see Chapter 12). Anxiety

disorders are more common in women and in middle age. Lower rates are reported in young men and older people, although the low rates in people over 65 may be due to the greater difficulty in detecting anxiety with standard instruments in this population. Having an anxiety disorder is also associated with socio-economic adversity.

Panic disorder

Panic disorder is characterized by recurrent episodic severe panic (anxiety) attacks, which occur unpredictably and are not restricted to any particular situation or set of circumstances (although certain situations such as being in crowds may become associated with them). Panic attacks are discrete periods of intense fear, impending doom or discomfort, accompanied by characteristic symptoms: palpitations, tachycardia, sweating, trembling, breathlessness, feeling of choking, chest pain/discomfort, nausea/abdominal discomfort, dizziness, paraesthesias, chills and hot flushes, derealization (the experience of the world, or people in it, seeming lifeless), depersonalization (feeling detached from oneself) and fear of losing control, 'going crazy' or dying. Typically, the duration of a panic attack is only a few minutes. A complication is the development of 'anticipatory fear' of the ramifications of having a panic attack, with the result that the individual may be reluctant to be alone in a public place or away from home. Both current classificatory systems (DSM-IV-TR and ICD-10) stipulate at least three panic attacks in a three-week period should occur for a diagnosis of panic disorder to be made, where there is no discernible objective danger to the individual, with relative freedom from anxiety between the discrete panic attacks.

Of the general population, around 1% has panic disorder; women appear to be affected more frequently than men and the typical age at onset is 25–44 years. Panic disorder shows familial transmission which is unrelated to GAD. Sodium lactate infusion and breathing in carbon dioxide can induce panic attacks in susceptible individuals. Selective serotonin reuptake inhibitors (SSRIs) and cognitive behaviour therapy (CBT) (see Chapter 33) or self-help materials that draw on CBT principles are recommended first-line treatments. Tricyclic antidepressants (imipramine and clomipramine) may be helpful where SSRIs are ineffective. Benzodiazepines are not recommended due to the risks of tolerance and addiction.

Generalized anxiety disorder

GAD is characterized by generalized, persistent, excessive anxiety or worry (apprehensive expectation) about a number of events (e.g. work, school performance) which the individual finds difficult to control, lasting for at least three weeks (according to ICD-10) or six months or longer (according to DSM-IV-TR). The anxiety is usually associated with subjective apprehension (fears, worries), increased vigilance, feeling restless and on edge, sleeping difficulties (initial/middle insomnia, fatigue on waking), motor tension (tremor, hyperactive deep reflexes) and autonomic hyperactivity (tachycardia, tachypnoea, dilated pupils). GAD often runs a prolonged course, fluctuating in severity over time.

GAD occurs in 2–4% of the general population, usually begins in early adult life and affects women more frequently than men. Men and individuals with stable premorbid adjustment do better. It often occurs comorbidly with other anxiety disorders, depression, alcohol and drug abuse.

Aetiological factors include a genetic predisposition, childhood experiences characterized by separations, demands for high achievement and excess conformity, current stressful life-events and biological factors (dysfunction of autonomic nervous system reflecting increased sympathetic tone or parasympathetic abnormalities). Several psychophysiological measures are increased in GAD, including pulse, skin conduction, forearm blood flow and muscular tension (measured by an electromyogram [EMG]). On the electroencephalograph (EEG), the alpha rhythm is decreased.

Differential diagnoses include withdrawal from drugs or alcohol, excessive caffeine consumption, depression, schizophrenia and organic causes such as thyrotoxicosis, parathyroid disease, hypoglycaemia, phaeochromocytoma and carcinoid syndrome.

As recommended for panic disorder, self-help, CBT and SSRIs are the recommended first-line treatments. CBT for GAD seeks to identify morbid anticipatory thoughts and replace them with more realistic cognitions, and teach distraction techniques, breathing and relaxation exercises. Benzodiazepines should not usually be used beyond 2–4 weeks. Other pharmacological treatments include SNRIs (serotonin-norepinephrine reuptake inhibitors), buspirone and pregabalin.

Phobic disorders
Agoraphobia

Agoraphobia accounts for approximately 60% of phobic patients seen by psychiatrists. It is more common in women, with typical age at onset 15–35 years. Agoraphobia often occurs concurrently with panic disorder and is characterized by fear and avoidance of places or situations from which escape may be difficult or in which help may not be available in the event of having a situationally predisposed panic attack. Diagnosis requires that anxiety is restricted to being in the following situations: crowds, public places, travelling away from home or travelling alone. Avoidance of the phobic situation should also be a prominent feature. The individual therefore avoids the panic attack-inducing situations or secures the presence of a companion. Some people with marked agoraphobia experience paradoxically little anxiety as they avoid all phobic situations. They may, for example, leave the house only occasionally to visit a very restricted number of places, avoiding supermarkets and all public transport. CBT is considered the mainstay of treatment and usually involves graded exposure to avoided situations (see Chapter 33), but SSRIs are also effective. Treatment response may depend on the patient's level of engagement with treatment and motivation to bring about a change in their situation.

Social phobia

Social phobia is increasingly seen as both common and treatable. Social phobia is equally prevalent in men and women. Onset is usually by mid-adolescence but affected individuals often do not present for medical attention for many years. The disorder is characterized by a marked persistent fear of social performance situations in which the individual is exposed to unfamiliar people or to possible scrutiny by others, and fears that he/she will act in a way that will be humiliating or embarrassing (e.g. blushing, shaking, vomiting). Generalized social phobia, with fear and avoidance of most social or performance situations, is more impairing than non-generalized phobia, in which only certain situations are avoided or endured with much distress. Management includes drug treatments, notably SSRIs, SNRIs, reversible inhibitors of monoamine-oxidase-A (RIMAs) and monoamine oxidase inhibitors (MAOIs); and psychological approaches (including exposure by systematic desensitization).

Specific phobias

Specific phobias are more common in women. They are characterized by fear of specific people, objects or situations (e.g. dentists, flying, heights, animals, blood). Treatment is typically by graded exposure therapy and response prevention, although short-term use of benzodiazepines may be helpful if the phobia is rarely encountered (e.g. when flying twice a year).

Obsessions and compulsions

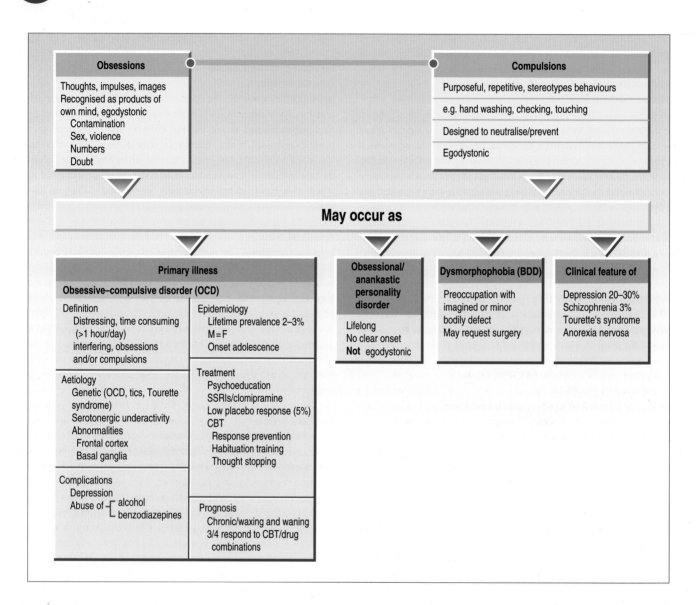

Definition

Obsessions are unwelcome, persistent, recurrent ideas, thoughts, impulses or images which are intrusive, senseless and uncomfortable for the individual, who attempts to suppress or neutralize them and recognizes them as absurd (egodystonic) and a product of his or her own mind. Obsessions may take the form of thoughts, images (vivid, morbid or violent scenes), impulses (e.g. a fear of jumping in front of a train), ruminations (continuous pondering) and doubts. Common obsessions include unpleasant thoughts of blasphemy, sex, violence, contamination, numbers and doubt. Obsessions should be distinguished from volitional fantasies (thoughts which are not displeasurable [egosyntonic]).

Compulsions are repetitive, purposeful physical or mental behaviours performed with reluctance in response to an obsession. They are carried out according to certain rules in a stereotyped fashion, and are designed to neutralize or prevent discomfort or a dreaded event. The activity is excessive and not connected to the triggering thought (obses-sion) in a realistic way. The individual realizes that this egodystonic behaviour is unreasonable. Common compulsions include hand-washing, cleaning, counting, checking, touching and constant rear-rangement of objects to achieve symmetry. Mental compulsions include praying, mentally checking and repeating thoughts. Rarer compulsions include arithmomania (counting), onomatomania (the desire to utter a forbidden word) and *folie du pourquoi* (the irresistible habit of seeking explanations for commonplace facts by asking endless questions). Inappropriate and excessive tidiness is another possible compulsion.

Compulsions should be distinguished from rituals and 'normal' superstitious behaviour (actions that have a magical quality and are culturally sanctioned, such as touching wood for good luck). If resistance to the obsessions or compulsions is attempted, anxiety usually increases until the compulsive activity is performed.

Mild obsessions and compulsions are common in the general popula-tion. They may also occur in depression, schizophrenia, Tourette's syndrome, puerperal illness (fear of harming the baby), anorexia nervosa, generalized anxiety disorder, dementia, temporal lobe epilepsy, Parkinson's disease, Sydenham's chorea (chorea associated with rheumatic fever), head injury and manganese poisoning. Recent evidence suggests that there is comorbidity between OCD and bipolar affective disorder.

Body dysmorphic disorder (BDD: dysmorphophobia)

This disorder, related to OCD (and also to hypochondriacal disorder), is characterized by a preoccupation with an imagined defect in appearance or, in the case of a slight physical anomaly, the person's concern is markedly excessive. Time-consuming behaviours include mirror-gazing, comparing particular features to those of others, excessive camouflaging tactics to hide the defect, skin-picking and reassurance-seeking; the sufferer may even request surgery.

Anankastic (obsessive-compulsive) personality disorder

Characteristic features include rigidity of thinking, perfectionism, orderliness and moralistic preoccupation with rules, excessive cleanliness and a tendency to hoard. These are egosyntonic life traits with no obvious onset. The perfectionism may interfere with the subject's ability to complete tasks and objectively high standards are seldom achieved. Subjects are often emotionally cold.

Obsessive–compulsive disorder

Clinical characteristics

OCD is characterized by egodystonic, time-consuming (>1 hour/day) obsessions and/or compulsions. A diagnosis of OCD (according to ICD-10) requires that obsessions or compulsives are present on most days for at least two weeks, that they are a source of distress and interfere with activities. Avoidance of stimuli or activities that trigger obsessive–compulsive symptoms is very common. Resistance is characteristic, but may not persist. Onset is usually during adolescence.

OCD can be divided into four subtypes. (1) The most frequent obsessions are concerned with contamination (43%); hand-washing is found in most studies to be the commonest compulsion (85%). (2) Checking compulsions are carried out in response to obsessional thoughts about potential harm (e.g. from leaving the gas on). (3) Pure obsessions (approximately 25% of OCD patients report obsessions without overt compulsive acts). (4) Hoarding (the acquisition of, and difficulty discarding, items that appear worthless to others). People who exhibit the hoarding subtype are particularly likely to have comorbid anxiety and depression.

Complications include depression and abuse of anxiolytics or alcohol. Severe OCD can lead to as much distress and functional impairment as psychotic illness.

Epidemiology

The lifetime prevalence in the general population is 2–3%. Men and women are affected equally.

Aetiology

In many patients there are genetic influences with a positive family history (50% of cases) of OCD. People with OCD are also more likely to have a family history of tics or Tourette's syndrome. Individual patterns of information-processing are crucial; a fundamental problem appears to be an inability to inhibit or suppress inappropriate mental or physical acts.

Biochemical abnormalities (especially involving serotonin) are now thought to be important in the pathophysiology of OCD. Brain neuroimaging techniques have shown functional abnormalities in the frontal cortex and basal ganglia. Earlier theories of aetiology include those derived from psychoanalytic thinking, which postulated that it represented a defence against cruel and aggressive fantasies; that is, filling the mind with obsessional thoughts to prevent undesirable ideas from entering consciousness. It was also thought to be a defensive regression to a pregenital anal–erotic stage of development. Behaviourists proposed that compulsive behaviour was learned and maintained by operant conditioning processes, the anxiety reduction following the compulsive behaviour strengthening, and ultimately increasing, the need to perform the compulsion in response to an obsessional thought.

Management

Psychoeducation about OCD helps people understand their disorder. Externalization of OCD (i.e. giving it a name) gives this distressing part of their personality another entity, which can be counteracted. It is now generally agreed that the combination of CBT and medication is the best treatment.

CBT involves exposure followed by response prevention (ERP) and may include habituation training for obsessions. During ERP the patient is instructed to desist from performing the unwanted compulsive behaviour (e.g. repeated hand-washing) while simultaneously being exposed to a situation (e.g. wiping a lavatory seat) which is likely to increase the need to perform it. Habituation training involves repeated exposure to obsessional thoughts (e.g. the patient listens to a cassette tape continuously repeating his or her obsessional thoughts) without allowing them to be neutralized until the individual habituates and the anxiety decreases. The opposite of habituation training is thought-stopping (well known, but less effective), during which the patient is encouraged to relax and ruminate until the obsessions are uppermost in his/her mind. The therapist then shouts 'Stop!' and the patient tries to stop ruminating. CBT can be delivered as self-help, group or individual therapy.

Drug treatment is with antidepressants, which act specifically on serotonin, such as selective serotonin reuptake inhibitors (SSRIs) and clomipramine. These drugs are effective even in the absence of coexistent depressive symptomatology. Neuroimaging studies show that similar changes in the caudate nucleus occur in response to both CBT and to SSRIs. Overall response to CBT and/or drugs is about 75%; in contrast, placebo responses in clinical trials are low (5%). The augmentation of an SSRI by antipsychotics may be useful in the treatment of both obsessions and compulsions. SSRIs and CBT are also effective in the treatment of BDD. Psychosurgery (cingulotomy, capsulotomy) is very rarely used, but may be effective in the most severe and treatment-resistant cases. Deep brain stimulation (see Chapter 37) has been used successfully recently but in a small select number of patients.

Course and prognosis

OCD is chronic, with waxing and waning of symptoms. Patients with prominent compulsions and those with comorbid tic disorders, persistent life stresses or premorbid anankastic personality fare worst. Traditionally, OCD was thought to carry a low risk of suicide; recent research contradicts this.

13 Eating disorders

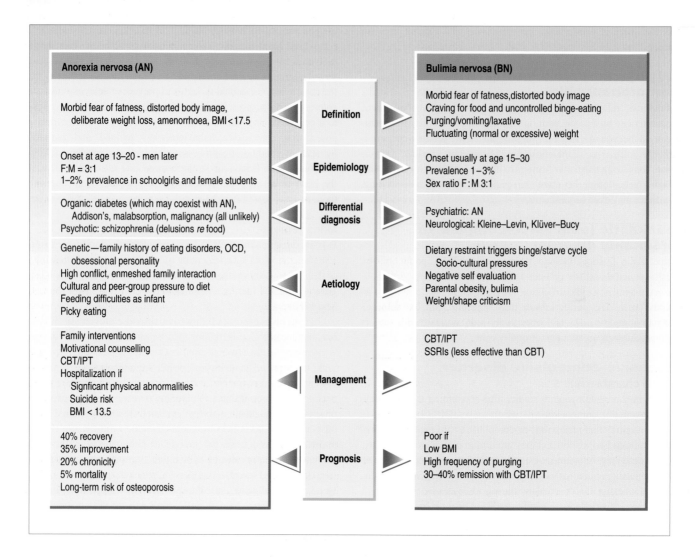

Anorexia nervosa (AN)

Definition — Morbid fear of fatness, distorted body image, deliberate weight loss, amenorrhoea, BMI < 17.5

Epidemiology — Onset at age 13–20 - men later / F:M = 3:1 / 1–2% prevalence in schoolgirls and female students

Differential diagnosis — Organic: diabetes (which may coexist with AN), Addison's, malabsorption, malignancy (all unlikely) / Psychotic: schizophrenia (delusions *re* food)

Aetiology — Genetic—family history of eating disorders, OCD, obsessional personality / High conflict, enmeshed family interaction / Cultural and peer-group pressure to diet / Feeding difficulties as infant / Picky eating

Management — Family interventions / Motivational counselling / CBT/IPT / Hospitalization if — Signficant physical abnormalities / Suicide risk / BMI < 13.5

Prognosis — 40% recovery / 35% improvement / 20% chronicity / 5% mortality / Long-term risk of osteoporosis

Bulimia nervosa (BN)

Definition — Morbid fear of fatness, distorted body image / Craving for food and uncontrolled binge-eating / Purging/vomiting/laxative / Fluctuating (normal or excessive) weight

Epidemiology — Onset usually at age 15–30 / Prevalence 1–3% / Sex ratio F : M 3:1

Differential diagnosis — Psychiatric: AN / Neurological: Kleine–Levin, Klüver–Bucy

Aetiology — Dietary restraint triggers binge/starve cycle / Socio-cultural pressures / Negative self evaluation / Parental obesity, bulimia / Weight/shape criticism

Management — CBT/IPT / SSRIs (less effective than CBT)

Prognosis — Poor if / Low BMI / High frequency of purging / 30–40% remission with CBT/IPT

Anorexia nervosa (AN)

Diagnosis

Diagnosis of AN (ICD/DSM) requires the presence of: a morbid fear of fatness, deliberate weight loss, distorted body image, amenorrhoea and a body mass index (BMI, defined as weight [kg]/ht [m]^2) of less than 17.5. Amenorrhoea may be primary (in prepubertal girls) or secondary; vaginal bleeds may persist in women taking the oral contraceptive pill. In prepubertal boys development will be arrested, or post-puberty, there is loss of sexual interest and potency.

Associated features include preoccupation with food (dieting, often with specific fat and carbohydrate avoidance, and sometimes preparation of elaborate meals for others), vigorous exercise, constipation, cold intolerance, fear of sexuality, depressive symptoms and obsessive–compulsive (often perfectionistic) phenomena. Self-consciousness about eating in public and social isolation are often found. Sufferers usually fall into 'restrictive' (minimal food intake and exercise) or

'bulimic' (episodic binge-eating with laxative use and induced vomiting) subtypes. Emaciation is often disguised by make-up and baggy clothes. The skin is usually dry and yellow and the trunk and face covered in fine lanugo hair. Bradycardia, hypotension, anaemia, leucopenia and osteoporosis are common. Consequences of repeated vomiting include hypokalaemia, alkalosis, pitted teeth, parotid swelling and scarring of the dorsum of the hand (Russell's sign).

Epidemiology

Most people with AN are women (although the prevalence in men is increasing, with the female:male ratio approximately 3:1); 85% have an onset at age 13–20 years. AN is increasingly seen in children, where the sex ratio is nearly equal. AN in men has a later onset (typically 17–24 years). Prevalence rates of 1–2% in schoolgirls and female university students have been reported.

Risk factors

Female gender and a history of exercising regularly before onset are the most important factors predicting AN. Other risk factors include childhood feeding difficulties, picky eating, gastrointestinal problems, problems with sleeping, over-involved parenting, childhood perfectionism, obsessive compulsive personality disorder and negative evaluation of self. Risk of AN in unrelated to socio-economic class.

A genetic component is indicated by the higher concordance for AN in monozygotic (60%) than dizygotic (10%) twins, and a high positive family history of eating disorders, obsessive–compulsive disorders and obsessional personality. A desire to avoid the consequences of sexual maturity has been implicated.

Differential diagnosis

Includes organic causes of low weight (e.g. diabetes mellitus), which are not usually associated with abnormal attitudes to weight or eating. Diabetes may, however, coexist with AN. Psychiatric causes of low weight include depression (which may also coexist with AN), psychotic disorders with delusions concerning food, and substance or alcohol abuse. There is an important overlap between AN and bulimia nervosa.

Management

Management initially involves medical stabilization and exclusion of other diagnoses. Coexistent depression should improve with weight gain, even without antidepressants. Individuals with AN value their emaciated state and typically are ambivalent about treatment. A good therapeutic relationship and motivational counselling are important elements in management. For adolescents, family interventions are the treatment of choice. For adult patients with AN effective psychological therapies include cognitive–behaviour therapy (CBT), interpersonal psychotherapy (IPT), focal psychodynamic therapy and family therapy (see Chapter 33).

Hospitalization (sometimes compulsory) may be necessary if weight loss is severe and rapid, if suicide risk is significant or if there are significant physical abnormalities resulting from starvation or purging. At BMI <13.5 the risk of death from fatal arrhythmia or hypoglycaemia is high and inpatient treatment is indicated. In very severe cases, nasogastric feeding may be instigated without the patient's consent under the Mental Health Act. Specialist inpatient programmes typically provide a structured, symptom-focused treatment regime to achieve weight restoration. Throughout inpatient feeding, the patient's physical state needs careful monitoring.

Prognosis is variable. About 40% of people recover completely, 35% improve, 20% develop a chronic eating disorder and 5% die from AN. Osteoporosis is a long-term complication.

Bulimia nervosa

The diagnostic criteria for BN are: (1) craving for food and binge-eating (eating large amounts of food in a short period of time [e.g. >2000 kcal in a session]). (2) Recurrent inappropriate compensatory behaviour in order to prevent weight gain, such as self-induced vomiting; misuse of laxatives, diuretics, enemas or other medications (or omitting insulin in diabetic patients); fasting or excessive exercise. (3) Preoccupation with body weight and shape, and a morbid fear of fatness. Binge-eating disorder without compensatory behaviours typically leads to obesity.

Clinical features

These include normal or excessive weight (which often fluctuates), a sense of loss of control and the stigmata of excessive vomiting. Sufferers may describe a trance-like state during bingeing. Amenorrhoea occurs in 50% (despite normal weight). Hypokalaemia may lead to dysrhythmias or renal damage; acute oesophageal tears can occur during forced vomiting. Psychiatric features include intense self-loathing and associated depression. In 'multi-impulsive bulimia' alcohol and drug misuse, deliberate self-harm, stealing and sexual disinhibition coexist, with poor impulse control being the common pathology.

Binge-eating is common in adolescence; the prevalence of true BN is 1–3%, with a 3 : 1 female preponderance. Presentation is later than for AN (late teens or twenties).

Risk factors

Female gender and a history of dieting; negative self-evaluation, parental obesity and being subject to weight/shape-related criticisms are risk fact. There is an excess of alcohol and substance abuse, depression and BN in first-degree relatives.

Differential diagnosis

AN, affective disorder and obesity should be considered. Rare neurological causes of overeating include Kleine–Levin (associated hypersomnia) and Klüver–Bucy (compulsive orality and hypersexuality) syndromes.

Management

Management involves medical stabilization and psychotherapy (usually CBT or IPT [see Chapter 33]) to establish a regular eating programme, re-establish control of diet and address underlying abnormal cognitions. Antidepressants have an independent anti-bulimic effect, best established for fluoxetine (60 mg), but are less effective than CBT.

Prognosis

Prognosis is poor in patients with a low BMI and a high frequency of purging. The benefits of treatment are, however, reasonably well established, with CBT or IPT giving about 30–40% remission, gains which are typically maintained.

Obesity

This is defined as a BMI >30. Its prevalence is culturally variable (e.g. high in the USA). Mild to moderate (but not severe) obesity is commoner in women and with increasing age. Aetiological factors include weight-controlling genes (e.g. leptins), family and cultural norms, high availability of cheap calorific foods and a sedentary lifestyle. Management involves a behavioural and educational programme to re-establish sensible eating, and cognitive or supportive psychotherapy addressing secondary low self-esteem. Anti-obesity medications such as sibutramine (a serotonin and noradrenaline reuptake inhibitor) or orlistat (reduces absorption of dietary fat) are only of short-term benefit. Drugs that antagonise cannabinoid receptors, the activation of which increases appetite, have recently been developed. Surgical treatment (jaw wiring, gastric banding, resection or bypass) is indicated in severe (BMI > 40) and refractory cases.

Pica

Pica is defined as the persistent eating of non-nutritive substances (e.g. coal or soil). It is normal in very young children. It may reflect psychiatric illness in people with learning disability, autism or schizophrenia.

14 Personality disorders

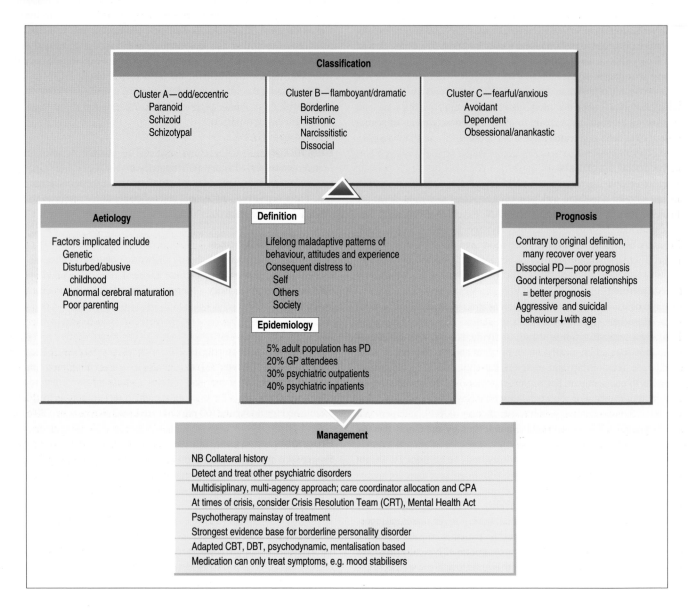

Classification

Cluster A—odd/eccentric
    Paranoid
    Schizoid
    Schizotypal

Cluster B—flamboyant/dramatic
    Borderline
    Histrionic
    Narcissitistic
    Dissocial

Cluster C—fearful/anxious
    Avoidant
    Dependent
    Obsessional/anankastic

Aetiology

Factors implicated include
    Genetic
    Disturbed/abusive
        childhood
    Abnormal cerebral maturation
    Poor parenting

Definition

Lifelong maladaptive patterns of
behaviour, attitudes and experience
Consequent distress to
    Self
    Others
    Society

Epidemiology

5% adult population has PD
20% GP attendees
30% psychiatric outpatients
40% psychiatric inpatients

Prognosis

Contrary to original definition,
    many recover over years
Dissocial PD—poor prognosis
Good interpersonal relationships
    = better prognosis
Aggressive and suicidal
    behaviour ↓with age

Management

NB Collateral history

Detect and treat other psychiatric disorders

Multidisiplinary, multi-agency approach; care coordinator allocation and CPA

At times of crisis, consider Crisis Resolution Team (CRT), Mental Health Act

Psychotherapy mainstay of treatment

Strongest evidence base for borderline personality disorder

Adapted CBT, DBT, psychodynamic, mentalisation based

Medication can only treat symptoms, e.g. mood stabilisers

Definition

Personality disorders (PDs) are deeply ingrained and enduring patterns of behaviour which represent deviations in a particular culture. They manifest as inflexible and unhelpful responses in a wide range of social and interpersonal circumstances and normally start in childhood/adolescence. They are not secondary to another mental disorder, but are frequently associated with subjective distress and have adverse effects on interpersonal relations and/or society.

The original distinction between PD (lifelong and not treatable) and mental illnesses (shorter duration and treatable) is now less clear. Recent evidence suggests that people can recover from PD and some effective treatments for borderline PD have been developed.

Epidemiology

About 5% of the adult population has a PD of at least mild severity, as do 20% of adult GP attendees, 30% of psychiatric outpatients and 40%

of psychiatric inpatients. While there is no clear consensus on which PDs are most prevalent in the general population, people with borderline PDs are particularly likely to present to A&E and psychiatric services (due to self-harming behaviours and severe emotional reactions to crises), while antisocial PD is common in prisons (Chapter 24).

Aetiology

As a rule of thumb, 'genes' and 'environment' contribute approximately equally to personality. Genetic influences are evidenced by monozygotic/dizygotic concordance; XYY individuals display increased criminality irrespective of IQ or socio-economic class. Poor parenting and an adverse environment early in life (during personality development) are implicated in both cognitive and psychodynamic theories. Cognitive theory suggests that people with PDs developed ways of coping with early life adversity (e.g. turning anger against oneself rather than expressing it if this could result in parental violence) which manifest as maladaptive traits later in life (e.g. problems in interpersonal relationships). Psychodynamic theories suggest that PDs result from disrupted psychological development due to an inability to form secure attachment to parental figures. Adverse intrauterine, perinatal or postnatal factors leading to abnormal cerebral maturation may predispose to PDs. An underactive autonomic nervous system has been implicated in dissocial PD. There is a strong association between sexual abuse in childhood and borderline PD.

Classification and characteristics

DSM-IV-TR groups PDs into three clusters. Patients (particularly those with severe PDs) may fulfil criteria for more than one PD diagnosis. The ICD-10 classification does not include narcissistic PD, but is otherwise similar to DSM (different names are given in parenthesis below). People should usually be assessed on more than one occasion, collateral history sought and comorbid psychiatric disorders treated before a diagnosis of a PD is made.

Cluster 'A' (odd/eccentric)

1 *Paranoid*: cold affect, pervasive distrust, suspiciousness of others, preoccupation with doubts about the fidelity or trustworthiness of friends or spouse, reluctance to confide, bearing grudges, reading negative meanings into remarks, hypersensitivity to rebuffs and a grandiose sense of personal rights.
2 *Schizoid*: social withdrawal, a restricted range of emotional expression, little interest in sex, restricted pleasure, lacking confidants, indifference to praise or criticism, aloofness and insensitivity to social norms.
3 *Schizotypal*: pervasive social and interpersonal deficits, ideas of reference, magical thinking, unusual perceptions (e.g. bodily illusions), vague, circumstantial, tangential thinking, suspiciousness, inappropriate/constricted affect, eccentricity and excessive social anxiety. Schizotypal PDs are commoner in relatives of people with schizophrenia.

Cluster 'B' (flamboyant/dramatic)

1 *Borderline (emotionally unstable)*: unstable and intense interpersonal relationships, self-image and affect; self-damaging impulsivity (spending, sex, substance abuse, reckless driving, binge-eating), identity confusion, chronic anhedonia, recurrent suicidal or self-mutilating behaviour, transient paranoid ideation and frantic efforts to avoid real or imagined rejection/abandonment. Bipolar affective disorders appear to be more common among people with borderline PD.
2 *Histrionic*: excessive shallow emotionality, attention-seeking, suggestibility, shallow/labile affect, inappropriate sexual seductiveness but frigidity and immaturity, narcissism, grandiosity, exploitative actions.
3 *Narcissistic*: pervasive grandiosity, lack of empathy and hypersensitivity to the evaluation of others.
4 *Dissocial (antisocial; psychopathic; sociopathic)*: persistent disregard for the rights or safety of others, gross irresponsibility, incapacity to maintain relationships, irritability, low frustration tolerance and aggressive threshold, incapacity to experience guilt or profit from experience, deceitfulness, impulsivity, disregard for personal safety, proneness to blame others.

Cluster 'C' (fearful/anxious)

1 *Avoidant (anxious)*: persistent feelings of tension and inadequacy, social inhibition, unwillingness to become involved with people unless certain of being liked, and restriction in lifestyle to maintain physical security.

2. *Dependent*: an excessive need to be taken care of, leading to submissive and clinging behaviour, fears of separation, difficulty in making everyday decisions without excessive advice, needing others to assume responsibility, difficulty in expressing disagreement for fear of loss of support/approval, difficulty in initiating projects (because of lack of self-confidence), going to lengths to gain support from others, constantly needing close relationships, undue compliance with other's wishes, unwilling to make demands on people and preoccupation with fears of being left alone.
3 *Obsessional (anankastic)*: see Chapter 12.

Management

Comorbid psychiatric illness and substance misuse disorders are prevalent in people with PDs, and their detection and treatment are a priority. Structure, consistency and clear boundaries (i.e. agreement of behaviour that is acceptable and unacceptable) are critical. Multidisciplinary and multi-agency work is often required. Admission to hospital, day hospital care or crisis team during periods of crisis may be necessary.

Supportive treatment is often delivered through allocation of a care coordinator (see Chapter 38). In people with borderline PD, threats and acts of deliberate self-harm and suicide can be difficult and time-consuming. Most people with PDs have a reduced ability to cope with everyday problems, so help with securing housing and other social matters may be required. A range of psychological individual and group therapies have been developed to treat people with (mainly borderline and dissocial) PDs. Adapted cognitive behavioural therapy, dialectical behaviour therapy (DBT) and mentalization-based treatments can be helpful in people with borderline PD (see Chapter 33).

Recent broadening of criteria for detention under the Mental Health Act (see Chapters 40 and 41) has led to the establishment of treatment centres in prisons and secure psychiatric units for people with dangerous and severe personality disorders who would previously have been managed by the criminal justice rather than health system. Psychological therapies require the cooperation of the patient, so motivation to engage in treatment is an important predictor of success.

Drug treatments are used to treat comorbid disorders. Drugs alone will not resolve the PD, but are occasionally used to control symptoms. Mood stabilizing agents may lessen episodic behavioural lack of control and aggression in borderline and antisocial PDs, and SSRIs are occasionally used to control impulsivity. Antidepressants may increase instability, however, so should be used with caution.

Prognosis

In general, individuals with PDs show decreased aggressive behaviour with age, although the ability to form successful relationships remains poor. Borderline PD carries a relatively favourable prognosis, with clinical recovery in over 50% at 10–25-year follow-up; schizoid and schizotypal patients tend to remain isolated. Dissocial PD carries a particularly poor prognosis. Certain individuals with PDs may relieve subjective discomfort by abusing alcohol and psychoactive substances, resulting in dependence and increased risk of accidental death. There is an increased risk of suicide in people with PDs; 30–60% of completed suicides have evidence of a PD.

Obsessional PDs are at high risk of progression to obsessive compulsive disorder or depression. Paranoid and schizotypal PD may progress to psychosis. Schizoid PD does not predispose to schizophrenia. Some PDs may confer susceptibility to physical illness (e.g. obsessional PD and duodenal ulcer).

15 Psychosexual disorders

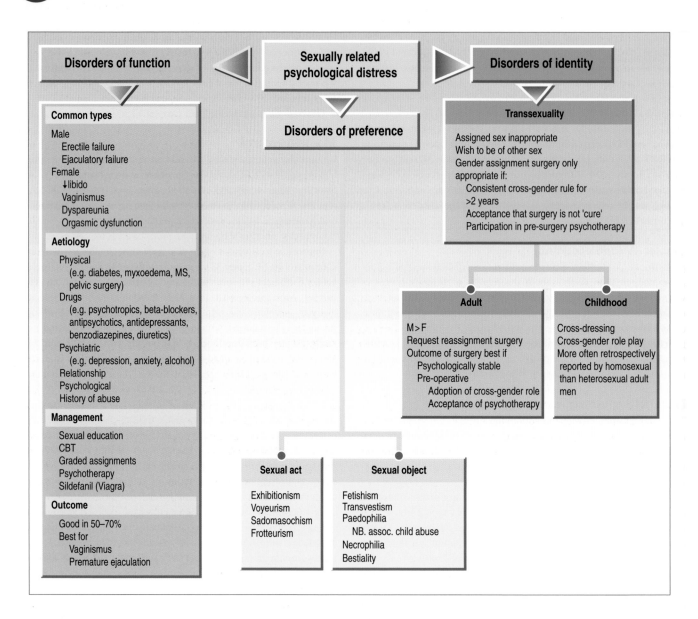

The range of sexual behaviour is extremely wide, with concepts of normality being socially or legally, rather than physiologically, determined. Moral and legal objections to some forms of sexual behaviour and an increasing awareness of the seriousness of sexually transmitted infections – particularly the human immunodeficiency virus (HIV) – and of what might be expected from a sexual relationship have encouraged the increasing medicalization of sexuality. Current psychiatric classifications (DSM-IV-TR, ICD-10) emphasize that sexual disorders have an element of psychological distress rather than being defined by behaviour alone. They can be divided into disorders of *sexual function*, *preference* and *identity*.

Sexual dysfunctions

Some degree of sexual dissatisfaction is present in as many as 20% of women and 30% of men. The commonest problems identified in both surveys and referrals to sexual disorder clinics are failure of erection

and/or ejaculation in men. In women they are low sexual interest, inability to allow penetration (vaginismus), pain on intercourse (dyspareunia), lack of sexual enjoyment and orgasmic dysfunction.

Assessment involves detailed history-taking from, and examination of, both partners in order to identify the nature of the problem, its duration, the couple's knowledge of and attitudes to sex and the reasons why help is currently being sought. Aetiological factors to be considered in the initial assessment include psychological factors, recent life-events, specific medical and psychiatric conditions (and their treatment), past sexual abuse and/or a poor general relationship with the sexual partner. Physical conditions impeding sexual function include neurological conditions (e.g. multiple sclerosis), diabetes, myxoedema and pelvic surgery. Sexual dysfunction may be induced by several prescribed drugs including beta-blockers, diuretics, antipsychotics, benzodiazepines and antidepressants, as well as recreational drug misuse, particularly involving the opiates. Sexual function is often impaired in depression (where loss of libido may reflect generalized anhedonia), alcohol dependence or misuse, and anxiety states, and may also be a manifestation of poor psychological adjustment to surgery (particularly mastectomy, colostomy or amputation).

Management increasingly involves a combination of medical and psychological interventions, including treatment of underlying medical or psychiatric conditions and 'couple therapy'. Until recently, physical treatments for erectile dysfunction in men involved intracavernosal use of drugs (prostaglandins, phentolamine), mechanical devices (vacuum pumps, penile bands), oral yohimbine or (rarely) surgical implants. Oral phosphodiesterase inhibitors such as sildefanil (Viagra) have largely superseded these interventions as the drug of choice for treatment for erectile dysfunction. Low-dose antidepressant drugs, which have a side-effect of delaying time to ejaculation, are also commonly prescribed to men with premature ejaculation.

Psychological treatments are essentially cognitive–behavioural and aim to facilitate communication, decrease anxiety about performance failure and identify and explore underlying developmental and personality problems. There is also an important role for sexual education, particularly dispelling myths about what is considered appropriate or normal sexual behaviour. This may include traditional sex therapy which (irrespective of the presenting dysfunction) involves the setting of a hierarchy of sexual 'assignments', structured on behavioural principles. The outcome is good in 50–70% of cases, with best results being for premature ejaculation in men and vaginismus in women. Other favourable prognostic factors include a good quality of general relationship, high motivation and early progress within treatment.

Disorders of sexual preference

The paraphilias may be classified into those where the primary deviation is the focus for the person's initial sexual arousal (rather than the subsequent sexual act) and those where it lies in the nature of the preferred sexual act itself. They are much commoner in men than in women.

It should be noted in this context that homosexuality is not considered a disorder of sexual preference. Subjects who are dissatisfied or unhappy with their sexual orientation are almost always so because of disapproval (e.g. by families or religious groups) or discrimination in society.

Variations of the sexual object include *paedophilia* (sexual activity or fantasy involving children); *fetishism* (where the object of sexual arousal is an inanimate object [e.g. an item of clothing or a non-genital body part]); *transvestism* (where sexual arousal is obtained by cross-dressing); and, more rarely, *bestiality* (sexual activity with animals) and *necrophilia* (intercourse with a corpse). Paedophilia is particularly important because of its link with child pornography and abuse (see Chapter 19). The aetiology of these conditions is unclear; management usually involves behaviour therapy (which may involve elements of aversion therapy and of conditioning more appropriate responses). Antiandrogens are sometimes used in paedophilia to help (usually) men reduce or control their sexual desire.

Variations of the sexual act involve the induction of both sexual arousal and (usually) orgasm by specific actions. Almost all people presenting to the courts or for psychiatric treatment with such variations are men. The commonest form is *exhibitionism* (indecent exposure) in which genital exposure is accompanied by emotional tension and excitement as well as sexual arousal. Exhibitionists make up one-quarter of the sexual offences dealt with by the courts, with psychiatric referral usually arising from this route. Exhibitionists fall into two main groups: those with aggressive personality traits or antisocial personality disorders (see Chapter 14) and in whom the act frequently involves masturbation; and those of inhibited temperament, where the exposed penis is often flaccid. Treatment may include psychodynamic, behavioural and hormonal (antiandrogen) components.

Other relatively common variations of the sexual act include *voyeurism* (observing sexual acts), *frotteurism* (rubbing the genitalia against a stranger in a crowded place) and *sadomasochism* (inflicting pain on others [sadism] or having it inflicted on oneself [masochism]). There are no systematic trials of treatment, although behavioural techniques are often used.

Disorders of sexual identity

This involves a strong wish to be of the other sex and a conviction that one's biological sex is inappropriate. It often begins in childhood, when it is characterized by cross-dressing, taking cross-gender roles in games and fantasy, and an attraction for pastimes usually regarded as more appropriate for children of the opposite sex. Gender atypical behaviours in boys are common, but they usually disappear as they are discouraged at school and by parents. Most boys who show gender atypical behaviour grow up to be straight, although adult homosexual men are more likely to report gender atypical behaviour in childhood than heterosexual men. Boys with clinical disorders of sexual identity do not regard themselves as homosexual as they grow up but rather as a woman (in a man's body) who is attracted to men.

The cardinal feature of disorders of sexual identity in adults (*transsexuality*) is a clear wish to live as a member of the other sex, with cross-dressing reflecting this desire rather than for sexual excitement. Most adult transsexuals are men. Transsexuals usually seek gender-reassignment surgery (with associated hormonal treatment). Outcome following such treatment is best where the patient is psychologically stable, has adopted the cross-gender role consistently for at least two years prior to surgery, accepts that surgical treatment is not a 'cure' and is willing to participate in pre-surgical psychotherapy.

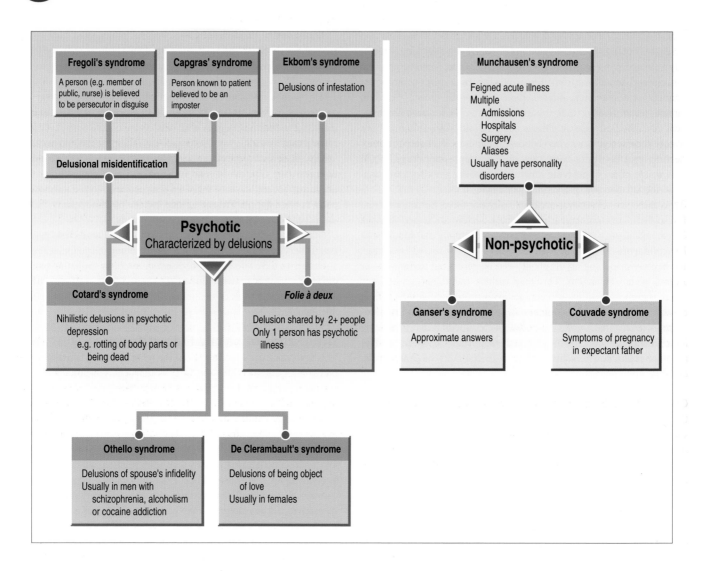

The features of the best described syndromes are summarized below. Although these syndromes have now been subsumed into the ICD-10 and DSM-IV-TR classification systems, their names are still in regular use. They can be divided into psychotic (characterized by delusions and hallucinations) and non-psychotic syndromes.

Psychotic
Delusional misidentification syndrome (DMS)
The best-known examples of DMS are the *Capgras'* and *Fregoli's syndromes*. Capgras' syndrome is characterized by a delusional belief that a person known to the patient (e.g. spouse or parent) has been replaced by an imposter who is their exact double. In contrast, the rarer Fregoli's syndrome involves the delusion that strangers or others the patient meets (e.g. nurses, doctors) are the patient's persecutors in disguise. The syndrome of intermetamorphosis is a variant of Fregoli's syndrome in which there is the delusional belief that there is interchange of mis-identified persons. The syndrome of subjective doubles is the delusional conviction that there are doubles of the patient's own self.

DMS may occur in schizophrenia, affective disorders and acute organic confusional states. Often an organic component accompanies these syndromes and sometimes their appearance heralds the development of dementia. Treatment is of the primary disorder. Risk of violence towards those who are the subject of the delusions should be assessed carefully.

Delusional parasitosis
Delusional parasitosis is also known as Ekbom's syndrome (although this term is also used to describe the neurological disorder of 'restless legs'). Sufferers (female:male ratio 3:1) believe that insects are colonizing their body, particularly the skin and eyes. Initial presentation is often to public health workers (with persistent demands for deinfestation), dermatologists or infectious disease physicians, with insistent, repeated and bizarre requests for investigation and treatment. Delusions may be circumscribed or part of a schizophrenic or depressive illness. Antipsychotics and/or antidepressants are the mainstay of treatment.

Folie à deux (induced or shared delusional disorder)

Folie à deux consists of a delusional belief that is shared by two or more people (usually within a family), of whom only one has the features of a psychotic illness. The pair are often isolated from others in terms of distance or due to cultural or language barriers. The delusion is usually persecutory or hypochondriacal, and the psychotic individual (principal) tends to be more intelligent and better educated than, and has a dominating influence over, the non-psychotic (more submissive) recipient(s). The diagnosis of the principal is most commonly schizophrenia, but may be an affective disorder or dementia; primary treatment is of the underlying condition. A period of separation of the involved individuals, followed by supportive individual and/or family therapy, may be helpful. *Folie à deux* is classified as Induced (ICD-10) or Shared (DSM-IV-TR) Delusional Disorder.

De Clerambault's syndrome (erotomania)

The patient (usually female) has the unfounded and delusional belief that someone (usually a man of higher social status) is in love with her. The patient makes inappropriate advances to the object of her passion and becomes angry (and sometimes violent) when rejected. The syndrome may exist in isolation as part of an affective (usually manic) disorder or, more rarely, schizophrenia. When men are affected they present a greater forensic problem. Management frequently involves hospitalization (sometimes compulsory) to prevent harassment or injury. Underlying conditions should be treated as appropriate; where no other underlying condition is identified, antipsychotics may be useful.

Othello syndrome (morbid or pathological jealousy)

Othello syndrome may complicate long-term alcohol abuse, and is also sometimes found in schizophrenia and cocaine addiction. The patient (usually male) is delusionally convinced that his partner is being unfaithful. He goes to great lengths to produce 'evidence' of the infidelity (e.g. stains on underclothes/sheets) and to extract a confession. Paradoxically, the partner is sometimes driven to true and actual infidelity. There is a substantial risk of violence (even homicide); thus, distant separation may be warranted and compulsory hospitalization and treatment are often necessary. It tends to re-occur with a new partner.

Cotard's syndrome

Cotard's syndrome is characterized by nihilistic delusions in which the patient believes that parts of his or her body are decaying or rotting, or have ceased to exist. Patients may also believe themselves to be dead or (paradoxically) unable to die and may therefore be eternally alive. Although the syndrome is almost invariably found in the context of psychotic depression, the nihilistic ideas themselves often have a grandiose flavour (e.g. the world will end because of them). Electroconvulsive therapy (ECT) is often required due to the severity of the associated depression.

Non-psychotic
Munchausen's syndrome

Munchausen's syndrome is termed Factitious Disorder in ICD-10 and DSM-IV-TR. It is characterized by deliberately feigned symptomatology, usually physical (e.g. abdominal pain), but can sometimes be psychiatric (e.g. with feigned hallucinations, multiple bereavements or sexual abuse). Occasionally the disorder can be by proxy, as when a parent fakes illnesses in a child (Munchausen's syndrome by proxy). These result in multiple presentations to A&E departments, usually to several hospitals, with frequent admissions often culminating in surgical procedures. Patients often use multiple aliases, are often of no fixed abode and usually have no regular GP. When discovered, the patients usually discharge themselves against medical advice. The syndrome characteristically occurs in the setting of a severely disordered personality. Management is difficult, although confrontation without rejection may prove helpful.

Important differential diagnoses are dissociative and somatization disorders (where symptoms are not consciously produced) and undiagnosed illness.

Couvade syndrome

Couvade syndrome consists of the experience of symptoms resembling those of pregnancy (abdominal swelling and/or spasms, nausea and vomiting, etc.) in expectant fathers. Anxiety and psychosomatic symptoms (e.g. toothache) are also common. The prevalence of mild forms is as high as 20%. The condition (which in some cultures is quite acceptable and may even be expected) is usually self-limiting and responds to counselling, but often recurs in subsequent pregnancies.

Ganser's syndrome (GS)

The central feature of this syndrome is the giving of approximate, absurd and often inconsistent answers to simple questions. The patient may say $2 + 2 = 5$, or, when asked the colour of snow, reply 'green'. The syndrome is also characterized by clouding of consciousness, true and/ or pseudo-hallucinations (visual or auditory) and somatic symptoms. In pure form, GS represents a dissociative reaction of defence against intolerable stress, and in ICD 10/DSM-IV-TR it is classified as a dissociative disorder. There may be an underlying depressive illness warranting treatment in its own right. GS is overrepresented in prison populations. Spontaneous improvement often occurs and is characteristically accompanied by amnesia for the abnormal behaviour. Recovery may be hastened by admission to hospital and psychotherapeutic exploration of underlying conflicts. Factitious disorder is a differential diagnosis.

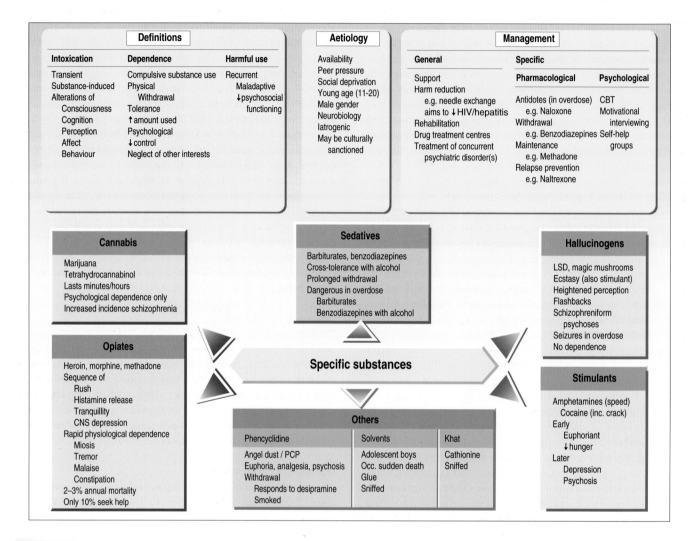

Definitions

Intoxication	Dependence	Harmful use
Transient	Compulsive substance use	Recurrent
Substance-induced	Physical	Maladaptive
Alterations of	Withdrawal	↓psychosocial
Consciousness	Tolerance	functioning
Cognition	↑ amount used	
Perception	Psychological	
Affect	↓control	
Behaviour	Neglect of other interests	

Aetiology

Availability
Peer pressure
Social deprivation
Young age (11-20)
Male gender
Neurobiology
Iatrogenic
May be culturally
sanctioned

Management

General	Specific	
	Pharmacological	Psychological
Support		
Harm reduction	Antidotes (in overdose)	CBT
e.g. needle exchange	e.g. Naloxone	Motivational
aims to ↓HIV/hepatitis	Withdrawal	interviewing
Rehabilitation	e.g. Benzodiazepines	Self-help
Drug treatment centres	Maintenance	groups
Treatment of concurrent	e.g. Methadone	
psychiatric disorder(s)	Relapse prevention	
	e.g. Naltrexone	

Cannabis

Marijuana
Tetrahydrocannabinol
Lasts minutes/hours
Psychological dependence only
Increased incidence schizophrenia

Opiates

Heroin, morphine, methadone
Sequence of
  Rush
  Histamine release
  Tranquillity
  CNS depression
Rapid physiological dependence
  Miosis
  Tremor
  Malaise
  Constipation
2–3% annual mortality
Only 10% seek help

Sedatives

Barbiturates, benzodiazepines
Cross-tolerance with alcohol
Prolonged withdrawal
Dangerous in overdose
  Barbiturates
  Benzodiazepines with alcohol

Specific substances

Others

Phencyclidine	Solvents	Khat
Angel dust / PCP	Adolescent boys	Cathionine
Euphoria, analgesia, psychosis	Occ. sudden death	Sniffed
Withdrawal	Glue	
Responds to desipramine	Sniffed	
Smoked		

Hallucinogens

LSD, magic mushrooms
Ecstasy (also stimulant)
Heightened perception
Flashbacks
Schizophreniform
  psychoses
Seizures in overdose
No dependence

Stimulants

Amphetamines (speed)
Cocaine (inc. crack)
Early
  Euphoriant
  ↓hunger
Later
  Depression
  Psychosis

Cannabis is the most common illicit drug used by the British general adult population (11% within the previous year), followed by cocaine (2.4%) and ecstasy (2%). In Britain, an estimated 500,000 people take ecstasy every weekend. Drugs are commonly used in combination.

In ICD-10, substance use disorders are classified according to (1) substance and (2) type of disorder. The latter include the following:

Acute intoxication: transient disturbances of consciousness, cognition, perception, affect or behaviour following the administration of a psychoactive substance (PS).

Harmful use: damage to the individual's health and adverse effects on family and society.

Dependence: physiological dependence includes a withdrawal state, tolerance (increasing doses of PSs needed for the same effect); and consequently the PS being taken in larger amounts or for longer than intended. Psychological dependence involves a sense of compulsion to take the PS, difficulties in controlling its use, increasing time spent obtaining, ingesting or recovering from the PS, persistence with PS use despite awareness of harmful consequences and a persistent but futile wish to cut down its use. There is usually a reduction or neglect of important social, occupational or recreational activities because of the PS use.

Withdrawal state: physical and psychological symptoms occurring on absolute or relative withdrawal of a substance after repeated and usually prolonged and/or high-dose use of that substance. Onset and course of the withdrawal state are time-limited and are related to the type of substance and the dose used before abstinence.

Psychotic disorder: psychotic symptoms occurring during or immediately after PS use, characterized by vivid hallucinations, abnormal affect, psychomotor disturbances and persecutory delusions and delusions of reference.

Amnesic disorder: memory and other cognitive impairments caused by substance use, most commonly alcohol (see Chapter 18).

Residual and late onset psychotic disorders: where effects on behaviour, affect, personality or cognition lasting beyond the period during which a direct PS effect might be expected (e.g. flashbacks).

Aetiology and management

Availability and peer pressure are key aetiological factors; there is a strong association with younger age (11–24 years) and male gender. Neurobiological mechanisms, iatrogenic factors (e.g. prescribed benzodiazepines [BDZs]), a desire for the pleasurable effects of substances and the pharmacological properties of the PS may all also contribute.

Substance misuse and psychiatric illness share several associations, including socio-economic disadvantage. Substance misuse can exacerbate psychiatric symptoms, commonly depressed mood, or precipitate episodes of illness (e.g. psychosis [Chapter 6]). Conversely, certain psychiatric symptoms, such as impulsivity or anxiety, may increase drug use, and patients with certain psychiatric diagnoses (e.g. dissocial personality disorder) are much more likely to take illicit drugs. Management of patients with psychiatric and substance misuse disorders (dual diagnosis) should ideally involve a multidisciplinary team trained to manage both disorders concurrently.

As well as being obtained illicitly, some PSs may be acquired legally from chemists (codeine), shops (solvents) or doctors (benzodiazepines, ostensibly therapeutically). In the UK, illicit drugs are controlled under the Misuse of Drugs Act. Drugs are classified as Class A (the most harmful, e.g. opiates, hallucinogens, injected stimulants), Class B (e.g. oral stimulants) and Class C. Cannabis is class C at time of writing, but may be reclassified to class B.

Treatment can be in residential rehabilitation, hospital and community settings. Medication has several uses: short-term treatment as antidotes in overdose and alleviation or prevention of withdrawal, or longer-term treatment as substance replacement therapy (e.g. methadone) or relapse prevention (e.g. naltrexone or acamprosate). Psychological approaches such as cognitive behaviour therapy, motivational interviewing (see Chapter 18) and self-help groups (such as Alcoholics Anonymous and Narcotics Anonymous) are effective. Infection (HIV and hepatitis C) is the greatest risk associated with injected drug use; harm-reduction strategies aim to minimize infection risk (e.g. needle exchange) and improve safety.

Specific substances
Opiates
Opiates include *heroin*, *morphine* and *methadone*. They may be smoked ('chasing the dragon'), sniffed ('snorting') or taken orally, intravenously ('mainlining'), intramuscularly or subcutaneously ('skin popping'). After an intensely pleasurable 'buzz' or 'rush' and release of histamine (itching, reddening of eyes), a sense of peace and detachment occurs, succeeded by central nervous system depression. Tolerance and withdrawal develop quickly. Ten per cent of opiate misusers become dependent, but only 10% of these ever seek help; 2–3% die annually. Of the remainder, 25% are abstinent at five years and 40% at ten years. Miosis, tremor, malaise, apathy, constipation, weakness, impotence, neglect, malnutrition and evidence of HIV and other infection (e.g. hepatitis C) are signs of chronic dependence. Early withdrawal symptoms (24–48 hours) include craving, flu-like symptoms, sweating and yawning. Mydriasis, abdominal cramps, diarrhoea, agitation, restlessness, piloerection ('gooseflesh') and tachycardia occur later (7–10 days). Opiate dependence may be treated by replacement with methadone (opioid agonist) or buprenorphine (opioid partial agonist), which are less euphoriant and have a relatively long half-life. Methadone, lofexidine and buprenorphine are used for detoxification; naltrexone (opioid antagonist) blocks the euphoric effects and so can help prevent relapse. Signs of overdose (often accidental) include miosis and respiratory depression and may require naloxone.

Hallucinogens
Hallucinogens include *LSD*, which produces psychological (e.g. heightened perceptions) and physiological (dilated pupils, peripheral vasoconstriction, increased temperature) effects, but not dependence. Rare adverse effects include 'flashbacks', psychoses and (in overdose) seizures. *Ecstasy* (MDMA, a synthetic amphetamine analogue) has mixed stimulant and hallucinogenic effects and can induce hyperactivity and potentially fatal dehydration (or hyponatraemia from resulting excess water consumption) and hyperpyrexia. *Magic mushrooms* (psylocybin) have effects similar to LSD but are less prolonged.

Stimulants
Amphetamines ('speed'), taken orally or intravenously, cause euphoria, increased concentration and energy, mydriasis, tachycardia and hyperreflexia, followed by depression, fatigue and headache. Acute use may induce a schizophreniform psychosis. Methamphetamine is chemically related but more potent, long-lasting and harmful; it can be ingested, snorted or smoked (as 'crystal meth'). *Cocaine* may be sniffed, chewed or injected intravenously. Its effects (restlessness, increased energy, abolition of fatigue and hunger) resemble hypomania and last about 20 minutes. Visual/tactile hallucinations of insects (formication) and paranoid psychoses occur. Post-cocaine dysphoria ('the crash'), with sleeplessness and intense depression, precedes withdrawal (depression, insomnia and craving). 'Crack' (a purified, very addictive form of cocaine) is smoked. The crack 'high' is extremely short and, on withdrawal, persecutory delusions are common.

Cannabis
The active compound of *marijuana* ('pot', 'grass', hashish, ganja) is tetrahydrocannabinol. The effects are psychological (euphoria, relaxation, well-being, omnipotence, hallucinations) and physiological (increased appetite, lowered body temperature). Substantial psychological dependence occurs. Adverse effects include conjunctival irritation, decreased spermatogenesis, lung disease, flashbacks, transient psychoses and apathy. Cannabis use is associated with increased incidence of depression and schizophrenia (Chapter 6).

Sedatives and hypnotics
Overdose may cause respiratory depression. *BDZs* produce dependence, withdrawal (including seizures) and tolerance. BDZ dependence is often iatrogenic, although BDZs are also common street (illicit/recreational) drugs.

Others
Solvents are typically sniffed, principally by groups of boys (aged 8–19 years) (a red rash around the mouth and nose may be a sign of abuse). Initial euphoria is followed by drowsiness. Psychological dependence is common, but physical dependence is rare. Chronic abuse results in weight loss, nausea, vomiting, polyneuropathy and cognitive impairment. Toxic effects (sometimes fatal) include bronchospasm, arrythmias, aplastic anaemia and hepatorenal or cerebral damage.

Phencyclidine (PCP; 'Angel Dust') is usually smoked. Its effects include euphoria and peripheral analgesia and impaired consciousness or psychosis, which may require antipsychotics. *Khat*, used particularly by men from the Somali and Yemeni communities, contains cathinone, an amphetamine-like stimulant causing excitement and euphoria. It is not a controlled substance in the UK. *Nicotine* – around a quarter of British adults smoke. Counselling, nicotine replacement therapy, varenicline (partial nicotinic receptor agonist) and buproprion (noradrenaline and dopamine reuptake inhibitor) may aid smoking cessation.

18 Alcohol abuse and dependence

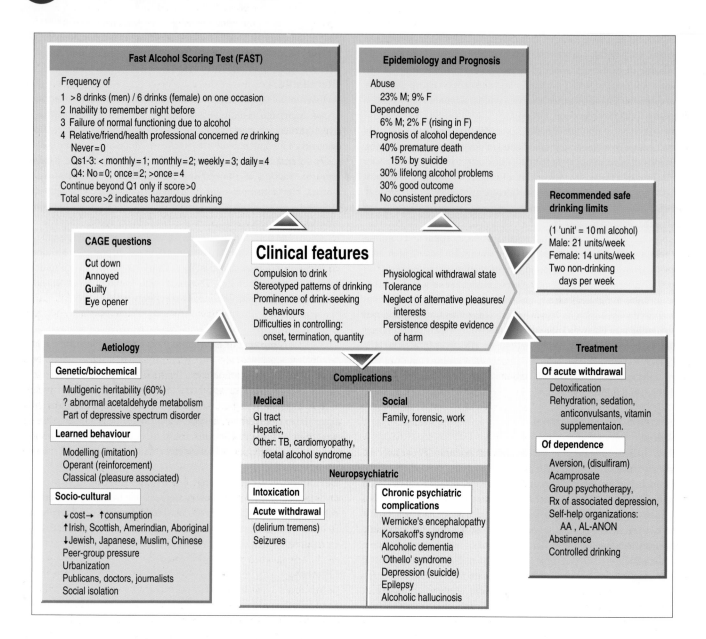

Fast Alcohol Scoring Test (FAST)

Frequency of

1 >8 drinks (men) / 6 drinks (female) on one occasion
2 Inability to remember night before
3 Failure of normal functioning due to alcohol
4 Relative/friend/health professional concerned *re* drinking
   Never = 0
   Qs1-3: < monthly = 1; monthly = 2; weekly = 3; daily = 4
   Q4: No = 0; once = 2; >once = 4
Continue beyond Q1 only if score >0
Total score >2 indicates hazardous drinking

Epidemiology and Prognosis

Abuse
   23% M; 9% F
Dependence
   6% M; 2% F (rising in F)
Prognosis of alcohol dependence
   40% premature death
      15% by suicide
   30% lifelong alcohol problems
   30% good outcome
   No consistent predictors

Recommended safe drinking limits

(1 'unit' = 10 ml alcohol)
Male: 21 units/week
Female: 14 units/week
Two non-drinking
   days per week

CAGE questions

Cut down
Annoyed
Guilty
Eye opener

Clinical features

Compulsion to drink
Stereotyped patterns of drinking
Prominence of drink-seeking
   behaviours
Difficulties in controlling:
   onset, termination, quantity

Physiological withdrawal state
Tolerance
Neglect of alternative pleasures/
   interests
Persistence despite evidence
   of harm

Aetiology

Genetic/biochemical

Multigenic heritability (60%)
? abnormal acetaldehyde metabolism
Part of depressive spectrum disorder

Learned behaviour

Modelling (imitation)
Operant (reinforcement)
Classical (pleasure associated)

Socio-cultural

↓cost→ ↑consumption
↑Irish, Scottish, Amerindian, Aboriginal
↓Jewish, Japanese, Muslim, Chinese
Peer-group pressure
Urbanization
Publicans, doctors, journalists
Social isolation

Complications

Medical	**Social**
GI tract	Family, forensic, work
Hepatic,	
Other: TB, cardiomyopathy,	
foetal alcohol syndrome	

Neuropsychiatric

Intoxication

Acute withdrawal

(delirium tremens)
Seizures

Chronic psychiatric complications

Wernicke's encephalopathy
Korsakoff's syndrome
Alcoholic dementia
'Othello' syndrome
Depression (suicide)
Epilepsy
Alcoholic hallucinosis

Treatment

Of acute withdrawal

Detoxification
Rehydration, sedation,
   anticonvulsants, vitamin
   supplementaion.

Of dependence

Aversion, (disulfiram)
Acamprosate
Group psychotherapy,
Rx of associated depression,
Self-help organizations:
   AA , AL-ANON
Abstinence
Controlled drinking

Definition and clinical features

The term alcohol abuse implies regular or binge consumption of alcohol sufficient to cause physical, neuropsychiatric or social damage. The conventional safe drinking limits are 21 units per week for men and 14 for women (a 'unit' of alcohol [10 mL, 8 g] representing roughly a small glass of wine, a pub single of spirits or a half pint of beer), with at least two drink-free days each week. Much smaller amounts may be hazardous to the foetus. In 1995, the UK government changed its guidelines to daily benchmarks (<4 units a day for men, <3 units for women), reflecting concerns about binge-drinking.

ICD-10 classifies alcohol use disorders using the same system as for other psychoactive substances (see Chapter 17).

Acute intoxication is characterized by slurred speech, impaired coordination and judgement, labile affect and, in severe cases, hypogly-caemia, stupor and coma. Differential diagnosis involves other causes of acute confusion, particularly head trauma.

Acute withdrawal usually occurs within 1–2 days of abstinence and is characterized by malaise, nausea, autonomic hyperactivity, tremulousness, labile mood, insomnia and transient hallucinations or illusions (usually visual). Seizures are a recognized complication. Severe withdrawal, or 'delirium tremens' ('shaking delirium'), occurs in 5% of withdrawals and has a mortality of up to 15%, partly as a result of other medical complications.

Alcohol dependence is a syndrome with cognitive, behavioural and psychological features, central to which are the compulsion to drink, preoccupation with alcohol, stereotyped drinking pattern, loss of the ability to regulate drinking, altered tolerance of the intoxicant effects of alcohol (initially increased but dramatically reduced late in the disorder), withdrawal phenomena and persistence even after attempted abstinence.

Psychotic disorders related to alcohol use include alcoholic hallucinosis (usually threatening, second-person voices in a clear sensorium) and pathological or morbid jealousy (paranoid delusions concerning infidelity). *Amnesic syndrome:* e.g. Korsakoff's psychosis (see below). *Residual and late onset disorders:* include residual depression and dementia.

Epidemiology

Prevalence rates worldwide vary widely and are related to overall consumption levels, availability and price. In the UK, heavy drinking (defined as 8 units/day for men and 6 units/day for women) is reported by 23% of men and 9% of women; younger people are much more likely to exceed safe limits. The prevalence of alcohol dependence is 6% in men and 2% in women. Rates in women and in adolescents are increasing.

Detection and screening

Neither alcohol abuse nor dependence is always clinically obvious. Their detection is crucial to enable appropriate counselling and treatment, and thus avoid long-term complications, and to avoid acute withdrawal in the context of unplanned abstinence (e.g. after surgery). General practitioners (GPs) and hospital staff should have a high index of suspicion in subjects with medical or psychiatric conditions associated with alcohol, and those with two or more drink driving offences. Many cases can be identified by documenting a 'typical drinking week'. Screening questionnaires are also helpful (e.g. the FAST [see diagram]). The CAGE questionnaire: – have you tried to Cut down drinking; have people Annoyed you by suggesting you do so; have you felt Guilty about drinking; have you needed an Eye-opener – remains widely used.

Collateral history can be revealing. Physical examination may reveal alcoholic stigmata, particularly signs of liver disease (jaundice, spider naevi, palmar erythema, gynaecomastia) and peripheral neuropathy. Macrocytosis without anaemia and raised γ-glutamyl transferase also suggest problem drinking. Carbohydrate deficient transferrin (CDT) indicates recent harmful use, as do high blood or urine ethanol levels without obvious intoxication.

Aetiology

Aetiology is multifactorial. Genetic factors have been implicated in animal and human studies, and by the striking differences in prevalence of alcohol dependence and abuse in some racial groups (e.g. high in indigenous Americans and Australians, low in Chinese and Japanese). These may be mediated by alterations in alcohol metabolism, those at low risk producing more (hangover-causing) acetaldehyde; 50% of Japanese people have an unpleasant 'flush reaction' on drinking alcohol due to a single genetic mutation in the acetaldehyde dehydrogenase 2 gene. Heritability (thought to be about 60%) appears multigenic. There is often a positive family history of depression. Social factors include occupation (high risk in the armed forces, doctors, publicans, journalists); cultural, particularly peer-group influences (low rates in Jews and Muslims, high in Scots and Irish) and the cost of alcoholic drinks. Behavioural models stress learning by imitation (modelling), social reinforcement, the association between drinking and pleasure (classical conditioning), and avoidance of withdrawal symptoms (operant conditioning). Risk increases in the presence of chronic psychiatric or physical illness, particularly if complicated by chronic pain. There is an association with mood and anxiety disorders.

Complications

These may be gastrointestinal, haematological and cardiovascular. The most dramatic **neuropsychiatric complication** is Wernicke's encephalopathy (caused by mamillary body damage secondary to thiamine deficiency and characterized by ataxia, nystagmus, ophthalmoplegia and acute confusion), which may recover with acute administration of thiamine, or develop if untreated into Korsakoff's psychosis (profound short-term memory loss characterized by confabulation). Other neuropsychiatric complications include peripheral neuropathy, cerebellar degeneration and erectile or ejaculatory impotence. Abuse of other drugs (particularly cross-tolerance with other sedatives such as benzodiazepines) is common.

Social complications include unemployment, marital difficulties, criminal activity, prostitution and road accidents. Alcohol is also often implicated in domestic violence, accidental deaths, suicides, up to 40% of A&E presentations, and homicides.

Drinking in pregnancy can cause *foetal alcohol syndrome.*

Management

Motivational interviewing (client-centred counselling that facilitates change by exploring ambivalence to seeking treatment, drinking cessation, or both) may help problem drinkers in denial achieve insight and a desire to change.

The first step in treating dependence is to achieve *abstinence* and this may first require acute *detoxification* which (like acute withdrawal) involves general support (adequate nutrition, reality orientation, good lighting) and measures to avoid specific complications. The latter include initially high but rapidly tailing sedation (benzodiazepine, such as chlordiazepoxide or diazepam, except in liver disease) to prevent seizures and control hallucinosis (this may also require antipsychotics); rehydration, correction of electrolyte disturbance, and B vitamin supplements. *Antipsychotics in DT ↓ seizure threshold (ddc drug)*

Abstinence may be a more realistic long-term aim than *controlled drinking*. Therapy to promote maintenance of abstinence or controlled drinking (i.e. within safe limits) can include psychotherapy, individually or in groups. Therapeutic aims are sustaining motivation, learning relapse-prevention strategies and developing social routines not reliant on alcohol, and treatment of coexistent depression and anxiety. Self-help groups (e.g. Alcoholics Anonymous) are helpful. Disulfiram (which blocks alcohol metabolism, inducing acetaldehyde accumulation if alcohol is ingested, with resultant flushing, headache, anxiety and nausea) and Acamprosate (which acts on the γ-aminobutyric acid [GABA] system to reduce cravings and risk of relapse) are licensed for the maintenance of abstinence in the detoxified patient. Naltrexone has similar therapeutic effects to Acamprosate but is not currently licensed for this indication in the UK.

Prevention involves reducing overall alcohol consumption; measures can include increasing taxation on alcohol and restricting its advertising or sale. Health education may be helpful, although evidence that it reduces consumption is not strong.

Prognosis

Alcohol dependence is characterized by periods of remission and relapse; 40% of subjects will die prematurely (15% by suicide) and a further 30% have lifelong alcohol-related problems. About one-third have a favourable outcome, although there are no factors that have been consistently found to identify a good prognosis.

Conduct disorders

Clinical features

Persistant antisocial behaviours
Violation of age-appropriate norms

Prevalence

4%
M:F = 3:1
↑ in low social class

Types

Socialized (peer acceptance)
Unsocialized (peer rejection)

Aetiology

Harsh/violent parenting
Family disharmony
Educational failure

Comorbidity

Disorders
　Hyperkinetic
　Learning
　Social-communicative

Management

Family therapy
Behavioural
Remedial teaching

Prognosis

Better if 'socialized'
2/3 persist in adulthood

Emotional disorders

School refusal

Not a diagnosis
Accounts for 1% school absences
Presents with somatic symptoms
Parental collusion common
Rx. Resumption of school attendance
　Graded
　Abrupt
Outcome
Good 60%
1/3 social difficulties / agoraphobia in adulthood

Generalised anxiety

Autonomic
　Palpitations
　Dry mouth
Psychological fear
Somatic abdominal pain

Phobias

Common in small children
Usually fear of
　Dark
　Strangers
Usually not clinically significant
2ndry avoidance may become pathological

Depression

Clinical features
　As in adults (see chapter 8)
Treatment
　Psychological therapy
SSRIs avoided
Completed suicide
　Rare
　Boys = Girls
Attempted suicide (DSH)
　F:M = 3.1
　↑ lower social class

Classification

Behavioural and emotional disorders
Social communication disorders

Sleep problems

Common in normal children
Night terrors in 3% age 4–7
　Assoc. tachycardia, tachypnoea
Aggravated by daytime stress
Usually resolve spontaneously
Nightmares respond to reassurance

Child abuse

Types

Physical
Emotional
Sexual

Vulnerability factors

Child
　Unwanted
　Low birth weight
　Handicap (mental/physical)
　Early separation from mother
　Persistent restlessness/crying
Parent
　Young and/or single
　History of abuse
　Unemployment
　Poverty

Signs

Unexplained injuries
Fear of parents
Failure to thrive

Consequences

Emotional, conduct and developmental discorders
Depression
Conversion disorders
Child-rearing problems
Personality disorder
DSH

Management

Detection
Report to agencies
　NB. Child protection register
Protection
Individual/family therapy

Psychiatric assessment of children

The assessment will involve interview(s) with the child and usually parent(s) (or carers) and teachers. In addition to usual history, ask about current behavioural or emotional difficulties (including mood, sleep, appetite, elimination, relationships and antisocial behaviours), school behaviour and academic performance, daily routine (including hobbies) and family structure and function (family interactions; past or current separations). Look particularly for signs of abuse or neglect, nature and level of spontaneous activity, rapport with interviewer, interaction with parent(s) and style of parenting. Physical, including neurological, examination is an important element of the assessment.

Classification

ICD-10 classifies psychiatric disorders specific to childhood into behav-ioural and emotional disorders (conduct, emotional, hyperkinetic, social functioning and elimination disorders) and social communica-tion disorders. Children also experience psychosis, anxiety, depressive illness or sleep disorders. In Chapters 20 and 21 we will consider these disorders and also the impact of child abuse. About 10% of boys and 6% of girls aged 5–10 years have an emotional or behavioural disorder, with the excess in boys due to higher rates of hyperkinetic and conduct disorders.

Conduct (behavioural) disorders

These are characterized by persistent antisocial behaviours that are major violations of age-appropriate social expectations; they include disobedience, lying, truancy, aggression, stealing, fighting, use of force and weapons, fire-setting and other damage to property. The prevalence

(4%) is higher in lower social classes and boys (×3). Low self-esteem and poor peer relationships are present in 20%. In 'socialized' conduct disorder, the antisocial behaviours are viewed as normal within the peer group and/or family; in the 'unsocialized' disorder, the behaviours are solitary, with both peer and parental rejection. The 'childhood onset type' and the 'adolescent onset type' refer to the onset as before or after the age of 10 years. *Oppositional defiant disorder* is a conduct disorder usually seen in children under the age of 10 years, characterized by persistent, negative, angry and defiant behaviours without more severe aggressive or dissocial acts.

Aetiological factors include family disharmony, harsh, violent, inconsistent parenting, and parents with alcohol dependence, antisocial personality disorder or depression. Conduct disorder is linked strongly to educational failure, and is often comorbid with hyperkinetic, learning or social communication disorders. Management usually involves a combination of family therapy, behavioural treatment of aggression, remedial teaching and the introduction of alternative peer group activities. Antisocial behaviours persist into adult life in two-thirds, and are associated with antisocial personality disorder in adult life. The prognosis is better in the 'socialized' group.

Emotional disorders

Emotional disorders are equally prevalent in boys and girls aged below 10 years (about 3%), but are more common in girls in adolescence. As well as anxiety and depressive disorders, which occur in all ages, ICD-10 includes diagnoses describing unusually severe or persistent emotional responses to normal childhood developmental phases, e.g. *separation anxiety disorder* and *sibling rivalry disorder*. Treatment involves a combination of behavioural and family therapy.

School refusal is not a diagnosis in itself. Child anxiety, bullying and difficult family dynamics are all common reasons why children refuse to go to school. School refusal accounts for 1% of school absences, with no gender or social class differences. The presentation may be with somatic symptoms (headache, abdominal pain). Three peak ages are recognized: aged 5–6 years (separation anxiety); aged 10–11 years (school transition); and adolescents (12+ years) (low self-esteem and depression). Parents (often overprotective with no excess of marital discord) are aware and often collude. Treatment is aimed at graded or abrupt resumption of school attendance. Outcome is good in 60%, although one-third have social difficulties and agoraphobia in adulthood.

Generalized anxiety, the most common emotional disorder in childhood, has autonomic (palpitations, dry mouth) and psychological (fear) components. Somatic symptoms, particularly abdominal pain, are common. Predisposing factors include the child's temperament and parental overprotection.

Phobias, particularly of the dark or of strangers, are common in small children and usually not clinically significant. When persistent and intense (often in response to parental or social reinforcement) the consequent avoidance may become pathological.

Depression presents similarly to the adult disorder. Treatment involves psychological therapies. The use of selective serotonin reuptake inhibitors (SSRIs) has been linked to the possibility of precipitating suicidal or aggressive behaviour in the young. Current UK guidelines recommend that these risks outweigh the benefits for most antidepressants (fluoxetine is an exception, although careful monitoring is still advised), however, experts may reasonably decide to prescribe them to under 18s in some circumstances. Completed suicide is rare in children, and equal in boys and girls. Attempted suicide is more common, girls attempting three times more than boys, and is associated with lower socio-economic classes.

Bereavement reactions are common, with similar symptoms and stages of grief to those experienced by adults. They may last for several months. Enuresis and temper tantrums in younger children, and sleep disturbance, poor school performance, acting-out behaviours and depressive illness in older children, may ensue. Where a parent has died, the surviving parent's coping mechanisms are crucial.

Obsessive–compulsive disorder (OCD). While minor forms of ritualistic behaviours and isolated compulsions (e.g. not walking on paving stone lines) are common in childhood, the prevalence of OCD as a disorder is estimated to be around 0.3–1%. OCD presents much as in adults and usually responds to cognitive behavioural therapy (usually requiring family cooperation). Fluoxetine may be prescribed cautiously.

Child abuse

Physical, emotional or sexual abuse or neglect can occur in all social strata and a high index of suspicion is crucial. Vulnerability factors in the child include being unwanted, low birthweight, early maternal separation, intellectual or physical impairments and persistent restlessness or crying. Young and/or single parents with their own history of abuse, socio-economic disadvantages (particularly unemployment) and unrealistic disciplining styles are particularly likely to abuse. Signs of abuse include injuries that are recurrent or lack a convincing explanation, and evidence in the child of withdrawal and/or fear of parents. Emotional abuse is an important cause of 'failure to thrive'. Signs of sexual abuse include age-inappropriate sexual talk, behaviour or play, secondary enuresis, sexually transmitted infections, waking up screaming in the night or nightmares during sleep.

Children who are abused are more vulnerable to emotional, conduct and developmental disorders later in childhood, and depression, personality, conversion disorders (e.g. pseudo-seizures) and child-rearing problems in adult life. Any suspicions should be reported to the relevant agency (Social Services in the UK, with police involvement as required), who will decide on the need for immediate protection and (in the UK) whether the child should be placed on the Child Protection Register (the means of supervising children considered at risk). Individual and family therapy may help with the emotional impact of abuse.

Sleep problems

These are common in normal children with night-time wakefulness in 20% and sleep-talking in 10%. Night terrors, in which children sit up terrified and screaming but cannot be woken sufficiently to be reassured, have a peak incidence (3%) at age 4–7 years and frequently a positive family history. They arise from deep (stage 4) sleep and are accompanied by tachycardia and tachypnoea. They are aggravated by daytime stress and usually resolve spontaneously. Nightmares (peak incidence age 5–6 years) that occur during REM sleep may be equally frightening and are also often stress-related, but the child can be easily woken and reassured.

Social communication (developmental) disorders

Autism

Epidemiology

Prevalence 4/10000
M : F = 3–4 : 1
↑ in Social Class I, II

Clinical features

Onset before 3 years
↓ ability to
  Relate to others
  React to change
  Language development
↓ IQ (>100 in only 5%)
Ritualistic/stereotyped behaviours

Prognosis

Poor (independent functioning in only 15%)
Better if
  IQ normal
  Speaking by age of 6

Asperger's syndrome

Similar to autism **but**
  Later onset
  Normal IQ
  Schizoid personality
  Frequent elective mutism

Hyperkinetic disorders

ADHD

Epidemiology

Prevalence 1% (UK); 7% (USA)
M : F = 3 : 1
Often associated with antisocial behaviour, language delay, clumsiness

Clinical features

Short attention span
Distractability
Overactivity
Impulsivity

Aetiology

Genetic
Social adversity
Parental alcohol abuse

Management

Behaviour therapy
Exclusion diet
Psychostimulants
  (e.g. methylphenidate)
Atomoxetine

Disorders of social functioning

Elective mutism
  Emotionally determined
  Language competence but no speech
    in some social situations
  Recovery by age 10 in 50%
Reactive attachment disorder
  Abnormalities in social relationships
  Associated
    Hypervigilance
    Fearfulness
    Aggression
    Failure to thrive
  Usually results from
    Neglect
    Abuse

Behavioural and emotional disorders

Enuresis

Definition

Urinary incontinence
  non-organic, age>5 years

Prevalence

↑ in boys
10% age 5, 5% age 10, 1% age 18

Aetiology

Positive family history
Unsettling family events
Development delay
Behaviour problems

Management

Exclude physical cause (e.g. UTI)
Parental reassurance
Behavioural
  Star chart, pad and bell, desmopressin
  imipramine

Encopresis

Definition

Inappropriate deposition of normal stool

Prevalence

2% boys, 1% girls at age 8

Aetiology

Anger, regression, emotional
  disturbance (NB. sexual abuse). Low IQ

Management

Ignore soiling
Avoid punishment
Star chart

Prognosis

90% improve

Hyperkinetic disorders (attention-deficit hyperactivity disorder [ADHD])

The core hyperkinetic syndrome is characterized by an early onset (usually 3–8 years) of short attention span, distractibility, overactivity and impulsivity which lasts longer than six months. It is more common in boys (male:female ratio 3 : 1), may be 'pervasive' (both at home and school) or 'situational', and is often associated with antisocial behaviour, language delay or clumsiness. It is less commonly recognized in the UK (using ICD criteria) (<1%) than in the USA (7%) (using DSM-IV-TR criteria), probably reflecting the UK usage of a narrower concept of ADHD.

There are several subtypes of ADHD: hyperactive, impulsive, inattentive or combined. ADHD frequently coexists with conduct disorder, anxiety, depression and specific reading retardation. Comorbidity predicts a poorer prognosis. Children with comorbid ADHD and conduct disorder are at particular risk of substance disorders in adolescence; severe forms are often associated with low intelligence, particularly in the context of brain damage (cerebral palsy, epilepsy). Other aetiological factors include genetic loading, social adversity, parental alcohol abuse, dietary constituents (lead, tartrazine) and exposure to tranquillizers.

Treatment approaches include behavioural therapy, which may be taught to parents to help them manage their child's behaviour (e.g. Webster-Stratton parenting programme), exclusion diets and prescribing stimulants such as methylphenidate (which is also available in slow-release form), dexamfetamine and atomoxetine, a non-stimulant drug that acts via the noradrenergic pathway. Tricyclic antidepressants, clonidine, buproprion and antipsychotics are also occasionally used.

Hyperactivity usually lessens by adolescence, although learning difficulties often persist and there is an excess of adult antisocial behaviour. There is increasing recognition that some childhood ADHD may be part of an affective (manic) disorder.

Disorders of social functioning

Elective mutism is a marked, emotionally determined selectivity in speaking, such that a child is able to comprehend spoken language and demonstrates language competence in some social situations, but fails to speak in others. Milder forms of the disorder are common but short-lived (usually at the beginning of schooling), while a clinically significant form is present in 1/1000. Affected children are usually very shy but stubborn and may have had previous speech delay; parents are often overprotective. Recovery occurs in about 50%; those not improving by the age of 10 years usually do badly.

Reactive attachment disorder is characterized by persistent abnormalities in a child's pattern of relationships with parental figures and in other social situations; it usually develops before the age of 5. There are usually poor peer relations, fearfulness and hyper-vigilance that do not respond to reassurance, aggression towards self and others, misery, withdrawal and, in some cases, failure to thrive. It probably occurs as a direct result of severe parental neglect, abuse or mishandling. It generally remits if the child is placed in a normal rearing environment with responsive, consistent parenting.

Other behavioural and emotional disorders

Enuresis refers to non-organic, involuntary bladder emptying after the age of 5 years. It can occur by day, by night or both, and is defined as secondary if there has been a period of urinary continence and primary if not. Prevalence is 10% at age 5, 5% at age 10 and 1% at age 18. The male:female ratio is 2:1. Aetiological factors include positive family history, unsettling family events, developmental delay and other behavioural problems in the child. Management involves the exclusion of physical pathology (especially urinary infection), parental reassurance and the institution of a behavioural programme (star chart and/or bell and pad). Tricyclic antidepressants are effective, but relapse is frequent when they are discontinued and behavioural methods and synthetic antidiuretic hormone (desmopressin) are often preferred. Ninety per cent resolve by adolescence.

Encopresis involves the deposition of stool in inappropriate places in the presence of normal bowel control. Most children are faecally continent by the age of 4 years. Prevalence is about 2% in boys and 1% in girls at age 8 years. Encopresis may reflect anger (with deposits positioned to cause maximum distress to parents/carers) or regression in children unable to cope with the increasing independence expected of them. Voluntary faecal retention with subsequent overflow is present in some cases. Physical disorder (e.g. Hirschsprung's disease) and other causes for constipation or pain on defecation must be ruled out. Encopresis is associated with emotional disturbance and other psychiatric disorders (although none is characteristic) and intelligence is usually average or below average. There may be underlying parental marital conflicts, punitive potty training and/or sexual abuse.

Treatment aims both to restore normal bowel habit and to improve parent/child relationships. Parents should be encouraged to ignore the soiling and in particular not to punish the child. More specific treatments include behaviour modification (e.g. star chart) and family therapy. Drug treatments are of very little use, except the use of laxatives if constipation is present. Ninety per cent improve within one year and almost all cases resolve by adolescence. Associated conduct disorder may, however, persist.

Psychotic disorders

Psychoses of childhood are rare. The most important are the childhood *schizophrenias*, which may be acute in onset (carrying a better prognosis) or have a prodrome of apparent developmental delay. As in adolescence and adulthood, there is a genetic predisposition and the presentation is with hallucinations, delusions and thought disorder, but with a greater preponderance of motor disturbance, particularly catatonia. Antipsychotics are the mainstay of treatment. *Mania* was thought not to occur before adolescence, but is now increasingly recognized in the post-pubertal years.

Social communication (developmental) disorders

Autism is the most important pervasive developmental disorder (PDD). It is present in about 4/10 000 children with a male:female ratio of 3–4:1 and is commoner in social classes I and II. The onset is before the age of 3 years and can even occur in the first few months. Three features are regarded as essential to the diagnosis: a pervasive failure to make social relationships (aloofness, lack of eye contact, poor empathy, etc.); major defects in verbal and non-verbal communication/language development; and resistance to change with associated ritualistic and/or manneristic behaviours. These may all reflect an inability to process emotional cues. Psychotic phenomena are absent. Affected children often develop inappropriate attachments to unusual objects, have a restricted range of interests and activities, exhibit stereotyped behaviours (rocking, twirling, etc.) and have unpredictable outbursts of screaming or laughter. Although the majority are of limited intelligence (IQ > 100 in only 5%), some autistic children have isolated skills (rote memory, computation). Learning disability, deafness and childhood schizophrenia must be considered in the differential diagnosis. Organic factors are strongly implicated in the aetiology; these include genetic loading and perinatal complications. Associated genetic disorders include tuberous sclerosis and Fragile X syndrome. Behavioural treatments, particularly operant conditioning, may reduce stereotypies and encourage more normal development and social functioning. Family support and counselling are crucial. Prognosis is poor, with persistent impairments in 60% and further deterioration in 20%; only 15% achieve fully independent functioning. Outcome is considerably better in those with a non-verbal IQ > 70 and if speech has developed by the age of 6 years.

Asperger's syndrome is a less severe form of PDD with later onset, normal intelligence and language development and schizoid personality. Pedantic speech and a preoccupation with obscure facts often occur.

Childhood disintegrative disorder (also called *disintegrative psychosis*) is characterized by normal initial development (to age 4 years) and the subsequent onset of a dementia with social, language and motor regression with prominent stereotypies. The aetiology includes infections (especially subacute sclerosing panencephalitis) and neurometabolic disorders. Prognosis is poor.

Specific reading retardation (SRR) represents reading difficulties that interfere with academic progress and are not accounted for by low intelligence, poor schooling or visual or auditory difficulties. Prevalence is between 5% and 10%, with a marked male and working-class preponderance. Neuropsychological testing often reveals perceptual and/or language deficits and there may be coexistent attention-deficit hyperactivity disorder (ADHD).

The psychiatry of adolescence

Mental illness			
Challenges	**Prevalence**	**Presentations**	**Assessment**

Physical growth
Moral development
Capacity to form relationships
Drives
    Sexual
    Aggressive
Autonomy
    Dependence vs.
    independence
	13% M, 10% F at ages
	10–15
	F > M 16+
	↑ with cannabis use
		Emotional upset
		Conflict with parents
		Delinquent behaviour
		Poor school performance
		Most with these indicators
		  not psychiatrically ill
			Allow for initial resentment
			Involve family
			Respect patient's
			  confidentiality

Commonest diagnoses (none specific to adolescence)

Conduct disorder	Disorders presenting in adolescence or adulthood

Norm-inappropriate
  behaviours
    Repetitive
    Persistent
    Violent
Comorbid conditions
  ADHD
  Depression
  Substance abuse
↑ risk of antisocial
  personality disorder
  as adult
	Mood disorders (mania 1%,
	  severe depression 8%)
	Stress-related disorders
	Anxiety disorders including OCD
	Schizophrenia
	Eating disorders
	Substance misuse disorders
	  Presentation and treatment
	    similar to adults
	  More focus on family
	  Medication avoided if possible

Adolescence starts with the onset of puberty and lasts until the attainment of full physical maturity. It encompasses sudden physical growth, surging sexual and aggressive drives (with associated uncertainties about sexual role, adequacy and identity) and the transition from separation from parents (and the associated dependence/independence conflict) to autonomy. Moral values may be expected to crystallize and self-esteem to grow. Conflicts between individual development and societal expectations may arise, and peer group pressures and influences are crucial. Added challenges include career choice and commitment to work. The capacity for lasting relationships develops in adolescence and any difficulties in forming relationships may emerge. About 13% of boys and 10% of girls aged 10–15 years have a psychiatric disorder; conduct and hyperkinetic disorders are commoner in boys and emotional disorders in girls. By early adulthood (age 16+), psychiatric disorders (mainly accounted for by anxiety and depression) are more common in women. No psychiatric diagnoses are specific to adolescence; most adult and child psychiatric disorders are seen, often modified by the patient's developmental stage.

Psychiatric assessment in adolescence

Common presentations of psychiatric disorder in adolescence include emotional upset, identity issues, conflict with parents, delinquent behaviour and poor school performance. Level of functioning and apparent 'disorders' must be set against developmental norms. Patients often do not acknowledge their own problems and referral by parents or schools may itself be a source of conflict and distress. Trust and rapport must be built up slowly in the face of resentment, suspicion and fear of being thought 'mad'.

Involving the family is important not only to provide corroborative evidence (the patient's own account often being inadequate or even falsified), but also to build up a picture of the family dynamics which may be crucial in both aetiology and management. A full account of earlier development is particularly important since many adolescent disorders have clear childhood antecedents. The diagnostic process is the same as in adults, and DSM or ICD classifications are used. Comorbidity is, however, even more common than in adults.

The patient's right to confidentiality must be respected, particularly in the context of sexual abuse. A parent has the right to give consent to treatment for a child under 18, provided it is in the child's interests. A child aged 16 or 17 is also presumed by law to be competent to give his or her own consent to treatment. Below the age of 16, children can give consent to medical treatment if a doctor judges they have the capacity to do so (see Chapter 39). If a parent refuses to consent to treatment that doctors consider to be in the child's interests, the child may be made a ward of court; the court can then overrule the parent's refusal. The Mental Health Act (see Chapters 40–42) may apply to a person of any age, but in practice children are usually treated informally with their consent or that of a parent.

Conduct disorder

Conduct disorder (CD) (see also Chapter 19) may emerge or worsen in adolescence. CD is characterized by the violation of age-appropriate societal norms. The behaviours are repetitive, persistent and often violent – bullying, mugging, shoplifting, theft, property damage or even armed robbery can occur. Substance abuse (see below), attention-deficit hyperactivity disorder (ADHD) and depression often coexist. Coexistent ADHD worsens the prognosis of CD. About one-third of adolescents with CD develop adult antisocial personality disorder, with continuing violent recidivism. Psychosocial intervention should be the first line of treatment, along with treating comorbid disorders. If problems are severe, medication may be used cautiously. Atypical antipsychotics (in particular risperidone, which is licensed for CD) may reduce aggressive behaviours, especially if there are coexisting neurodevelopmental disorders, such as autistic spectrum disorder. Selective serotonin reuptake inhibitors (SSRIs) may reduce impulsivity, irritability and lability of mood.

Eating disorders

Anorexia nervosa (AN) and bulimia nervosa (BN) are each found in about 1% of adolescents. AN has its peak prevalence in adolescence, and if mild may be difficult to distinguish from age-appropriate preoccupation with dieting. Adolescent-onset BN is increasingly common. Obesity is also common in adolescence (prevalence 20–30%) (see also Chapter 13).

Substance abuse

Experimentation with psychoactive substances (tobacco, alcohol, illegal drugs) is common in adolescence, reflecting both adolescent rebellion and the easy availability of the substances. Family and social adversity, vulnerable personality, peer pressure and associated CD or depression can contribute to the aetiology of adolescent substance abuse. The hallmarks of problematic abuse are abrupt deterioration in school performance (absenteeism, low grades, poor discipline), social difficulties (lawbreaking, fights, apparent personality change), lethargy, lack of motivation, slurred speech, drowsiness, lack of concentration and an unexplained deterioration in physical health. The patient usually denies any problems, and information from school or friends may therefore be vital. There is a strong link between mental disorder and rates of cigarette smoking, drinking and cannabis use among children aged 11–15; a recent survey found that over 40% who smoked cigarettes regularly had a mental disorder, most frequently a conduct or hyperkinetic disorder. Depression is frequent; the rise in adolescent suicide is largely accounted for by substance abusers and suicide risk must therefore be assessed.

Mood disorders

Mild episodes of depression (characterized by loneliness and low self-esteem) occur in 25% of adolescents and moderate or severe depression in about 8%. Depression is about four times commoner in adolescent girls than boys. Clinical features are essentially the same as in adults, but poor appetite, weight loss and feelings of hopelessness may be more prominent than overt sadness; sleep is more often prolonged than disrupted. Suicidal thoughts and minor acts of deliberate self-harm are common; actual suicide (particularly in boys and where there is coexistent substance abuse) has become more frequent in recent years and the risk must be considered.

Anxiety, eating disorders, substance abuse and ADHD all frequently coexist with depression in adolescence. Intervention may include family therapy and individual psychotherapy (particularly cognitive behavioural therapy; see Chapter 33). Antidepressants (see Chapter 35) may be indicated where biological features are prominent. In 2003, following concerns that SSRIs may increase the risk of suicidal thoughts and self-harm, the Committee on Safety of Medicines recommended that fluoxetine was the only SSRI with a favourable balance of risks and benefits for use in the treatment for major depressive episode in youths under the age of 18.

Mania has a prevalence of up to 1% in adolescence; the presentation and management principles are similar to those in adults (see Chapter 9). Substance abuse and schizophrenia are the main differential diagnoses.

Anxiety, stress-related disorders

Anxiety most frequently presents as overwhelming, non-specific worrying and repeated demands for reassurance. School refusal (as opposed to truancy) may arise from specific school-related phobias, anxiety or depression. Social phobias, characterized by avoiding contact with strangers, are also seen. Milder forms may respond to reassurance and advice (to adolescent, parents and school) on coping strategies; in more serious cases, response to relaxation therapy and desensitization is usually favourable (see Chapter 33). Anxiety may also arise in response to stress; presentations and management of acute stress reaction and post-traumatic stress disorder (PTSD) are similar to adults.

Obsessive–compulsive disorder (OCD)

Mild obsessionality is common in adolescence; true OCD may show prominent obsessional slowness and behaviour sufficiently bizarre to resemble schizophrenia. Resistance to the thoughts and behaviours may be absent. Treatment usually involves cognitive behavioural therapy and behavioural treatments (e.g. modelling and response prevention). Where psychological treatment alone is not sufficient, SSRIs are recommended, with careful monitoring for side-effects. OCD usually continues into adulthood (see also Chapter 12).

Schizophrenia

The peak age of onset of schizophrenia is in late adolescence. Presentation is usually with deteriorating school performance; clinical features are otherwise as in adult life. In younger adolescents, initial presentation is often with bizarre behaviour, social withdrawal and anxiety, with only fleeting first-rank symptoms. The differential diagnosis includes organic states, affective psychosis, drug-induced psychosis, adolescent crises and schizoid personality. Atypical antipsychotics and rehabilitation are the mainstays of management. Given the limited safety data on antipsychotic use in youth, clinicians should be vigilant for side-effects (see Chapter 34).

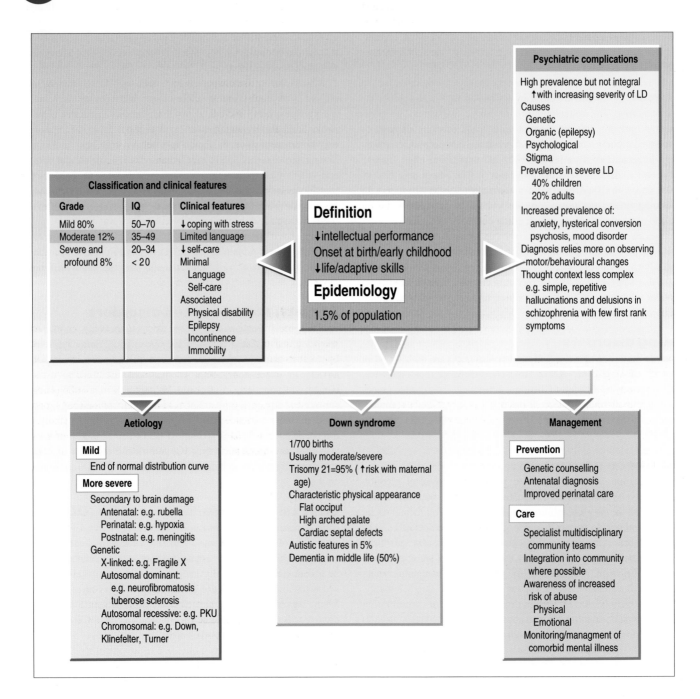

Classification and clinical features

Grade	IQ	Clinical features
Mild 80%	50–70	↓ coping with stress
Moderate 12%	35–49	Limited language
Severe and profound 8%	20–34 <20	↓ self-care Minimal Language Self-care Associated Physical disability Epilepsy Incontinence Immobility

Definition

↓intellectual performance
Onset at birth/early childhood
↓life/adaptive skills

Epidemiology

1.5% of population

Psychiatric complications

High prevalence but not integral
↑with increasing severity of LD
Causes
  Genetic
  Organic (epilepsy)
  Psychological
  Stigma
Prevalence in severe LD
  40% children
  20% adults
Increased prevalence of:
  anxiety, hysterical conversion
  psychosis, mood disorder
Diagnosis relies more on observing
  motor/behavioural changes
Thought context less complex
  e.g. simple, repetitive
  hallucinations and delusions in
  schizophrenia with few first rank
  symptoms

Aetiology

Mild
  End of normal distribution curve
More severe
  Secondary to brain damage
    Antenatal: e.g. rubella
    Perinatal: e.g. hypoxia
    Postnatal: e.g. meningitis
  Genetic
    X-linked: e.g. Fragile X
    Autosomal dominant:
      e.g. neurofibromatosis
      tuberose sclerosis
    Autosomal recessive: e.g. PKU
    Chromosomal: e.g. Down,
    Klinefelter, Turner

Down syndrome

1/700 births
Usually moderate/severe
Trisomy 21=95% (↑risk with maternal
  age)
Characteristic physical appearance
  Flat occiput
  High arched palate
  Cardiac septal defects
Autistic features in 5%
Dementia in middle life (50%)

Management

Prevention
  Genetic counselling
  Antenatal diagnosis
  Improved perinatal care
Care
  Specialist multidisciplinary
    community teams
  Integration into community
    where possible
  Awareness of increased
    risk of abuse
    Physical
    Emotional
  Monitoring/managment of
    comorbid mental illness

Definition

Learning disability (LD), referred to as mental retardation in current classificatory systems, has three main components: low intellectual performance; onset at birth or in early childhood; and reduced life/adaptive skills. LD is present in about 1.5% of the population, of whom 80% have mild LD, about 12% moderate LD and 7% are severely affected. Only 1% of the total is profoundly affected. The prevalence of LD has not fallen despite recent reductions in the incidence of severe LD. This reflects concurrent improvements in prevention (see below) and survival.

Classification and clinical features

LD can be conceptualized in terms of the primary impairment that causes it, the consequent disability and any resultant social handicap (including family difficulties). Intellectual impairment is classified as mild (IQ 50–70); moderate (35–49); severe (20–34) and profound (<20). Mild LD is not usually associated with abnormalities in appearance or behaviour; language, sensory and motor abnormalities are slight or absent. The problem is usually not apparent until school age. Adults with mild LD may have difficulty in coping with stress and often need support with more complex areas of social functioning, such as parenting and handling money. The majority are, however, able to live independently in the community and engage in some employment. People with moderate LD usually have limited but useful language. Severe and profound LD is associated with very limited verbal and self-care skills; associated physical disabilities/problems (epilepsy in 33%, incontinence in about 10%, inability to walk in about 15%) are very common. Communication may be facilitated by non-verbal techniques such as pointing or signing.

Mild LD is not usually associated with specific causes and represents the bottom end of a normal distribution curve for IQ; there is a considerable genetic contribution reflecting the high heritability of IQ in general. The close correlation between low parental and low child IQ is due in part to social and educational deprivation. More severe LD is usually related to specific brain damage. Causes may be antenatal (genetic, infective [e.g. toxoplasma, rubella and cytomegalovirus], hypoxic, toxic or related to maternal disease [toxaemia of pregnancy]), perinatal (prematurity, birth hypoxia, intracerebral bleed) or postnatal (infection, injury [particularly non-accidental], malnutrition, hormonal, metabolic, toxic, epileptic). Genetic causes may be chromosomal, e.g. Down, Klinefelter or Turner's syndrome, X-linked (Fragile X, Lesch–Nyhan), autosomal dominant (tuberose sclerosis, neurofibromatosis) and autosomal recessive, the latter usually associated with specific metabolic disorders such as phenylketonuria. Autism (see Chapter 20) is usually, although not invariably, associated with LD.

Down syndrome (DS)

DS is the commonest specific cause of LD, affecting about 1/700 births. The LD is usually moderate or severe, but mild in 15%. In 95% of cases there is trisomy of chromosome 21, risk of which increases with increasing maternal age (1/50 births with maternal age >45 years). In the remainder, DS is the result of translocation of chromosome 21 material; parents and siblings may be carriers. DS is associated with several physical abnormalities, including flat occiput, oblique palpebral fissures, small mouth with high, arched palate and broad hands with a single transverse palmar crease. Cardiac septal defects are common and used to result in high early mortality; nowadays they are often corrected surgically. Hypothyroidism is common. Autistic features are present in 5%. People with DS surviving beyond the age of 50 years invariably develop neuropathological changes akin to Alzheimer's disease which are visible on post-mortem; at least 50% have clinical dementia in life.

Fragile X syndrome

Fragile X is the second commonest cause of LD. It affects 1 in 3600 male and 1 in 5000 female births, accounting for 8% of males with LD. Physical signs include large head and ears, connective tissue disorders and mitral valve prolapse. Psychiatric features include abnormal speech, impulsivity and hyperactivity, hand-biting, hand-flapping, poor eye contact and unusual responses to various touch, auditory or visual stimuli. Four per cent have autistic features. Women often have less severe behavioural problems, and only a third have significant LD.

Psychiatric illness

Studies using appropriately structured interviews, detailed behavioural observations and carer interviews reveal that the prevalence of several psychiatric disorders (including behavioural disturbance) is increased in people with LD, especially those living in institutions, but is not integral to it. Making specific psychiatric diagnoses is, however, difficult (particularly in people with moderate or severe LD) because of coexisting language deficits. Behavioural disturbance is commoner with increasing severity of LD, occurring in up to 40% of children and 20% of adults with severe LD. This may include purposeless or self-injurious behaviour, aggression or inappropriate sexual behaviour (such as masturbation) in public.

Schizophrenia has a prevalence of 3% in people with learning disability and usually presents with simple and repetitive hallucinations and unelaborated, usually persecutory, delusions, which lack the complexity of first-rank symptoms (see Chapter 2). Rates of depression and anxiety disorders (including obsessive compulsive disorder and phobias) are also higher than in the general population. The diagnosis of depression rests more on motor and behavioural changes (reduced sleep, retardation, tearfulness, etc.) than verbal expressions of distress; similarly, mania usually presents as overactive and/or irritable behaviour. Dissociative symptoms are common. Psychological reactions to adverse life-events (such as bereavement) are often not recognized as such by carers. Psychiatric or physical health problems are sometimes not identified because symptoms are attributed to the person's LD. Genetic, organic (particularly epilepsy), psychological (frustration) and social factors such as stigma may all contribute to the excess of psychiatric problems associated with LD.

Prevention

Prevention of LD may be attempted before birth through genetic counselling and antenatal diagnosis; in particular, DS may be detected by amniocentesis or chorionic villus sampling, with the option of termination of pregnancy. Improved perinatal care reduces the risk of brain injury, and early detection of hormonal or metabolic problems (myxoedema, phenylketonuria) may allow treatment before LD occurs. There is some evidence that educational intervention in children of mothers with mild LD may enhance their educational performance (although not necessarily their IQ) and reduce the risk of conduct disorder.

Management

Most people with LD now live in domestic homes, usually with their families. Support is provided by primary care, educational and social services. Children with mild LD usually receive educational support within mainstream schools; as adults, they may need support to work in mainstream employment. Training may enable adults with moderate LD to work in sheltered settings; a small minority (with severe or profound LD and, usually, associated behavioural problems) need residential care. Specialist multidisciplinary community teams coordinate local services, assess and manage any concurrent mental illness, social skills and problem-solving training, and support with finances and accommodation. Treatment of mental illness is similar to that for patients without LD. Challenging behaviour is usually managed with behavioural therapy and changes to the individual's living situation and daily activities. People with LD need written information to be accessible (in a format the patient can understand). Those with more severe LD sometimes use Makaton, a communication system of signs and gestures. People with LD often face distress at the realization that they may not achieve full independence and that their parents are likely to die before they do, as well as issues around their sexuality. These are often difficult for carers and professionals to discuss. Sensitive but frank communication at a level the person with LD can understand is important. People with LD, especially those living in institutions, are at increased risk of physical, emotional and sexual abuse.

Cross-cultural psychiatry

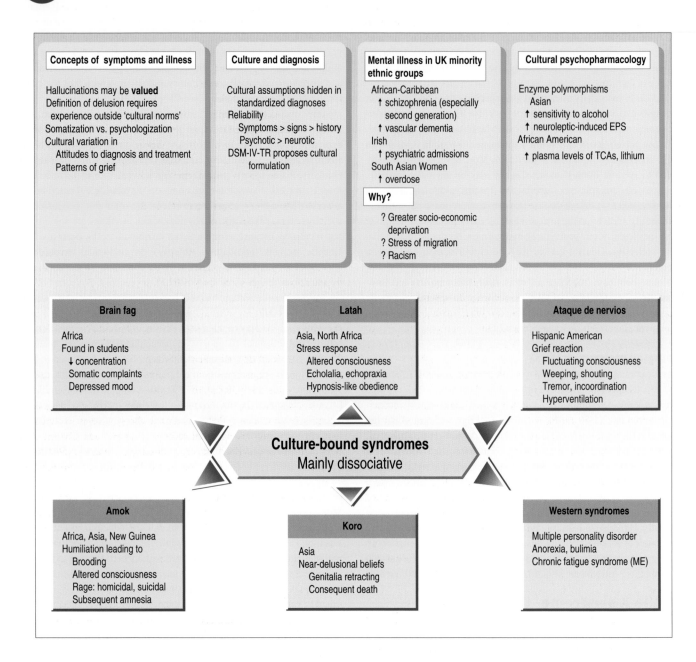

Concepts of symptoms and illness

Hallucinations may be **valued**
Definition of delusion requires
  experience outside 'cultural norms'
Somatization vs. psychologization
Cultural variation in
  Attitudes to diagnosis and treatment
  Patterns of grief

Culture and diagnosis

Cultural assumptions hidden in
  standardized diagnoses
Reliability
  Symptoms > signs > history
  Psychotic > neurotic
DSM-IV-TR proposes cultural
  formulation

Mental illness in UK minority ethnic groups

African-Caribbean
  ↑ schizophrenia (especially
    second generation)
  ↑ vascular dementia
Irish
  ↑ psychiatric admissions
South Asian Women
  ↑ overdose

Why?

? Greater socio-economic
  deprivation
? Stress of migration
? Racism

Cultural psychopharmacology

Enzyme polymorphisms
  Asian
  ↑ sensitivity to alcohol
  ↑ neuroleptic-induced EPS
African American
  ↑ plasma levels of TCAs, lithium

Brain fag

Africa
Found in students
  ↓ concentration
  Somatic complaints
  Depressed mood

Latah

Asia, North Africa
Stress response
  Altered consciousness
  Echolalia, echopraxia
  Hypnosis-like obedience

Ataque de nervios

Hispanic American
Grief reaction
  Fluctuating consciousness
  Weeping, shouting
  Tremor, incoordination
  Hyperventilation

Culture-bound syndromes
Mainly dissociative

Amok

Africa, Asia, New Guinea
Humiliation leading to
  Brooding
  Altered consciousness
  Rage: homicidal, suicidal
  Subsequent amnesia

Koro

Asia
Near-delusional beliefs
  Genitalia retracting
  Consequent death

Western syndromes

Multiple personality disorder
Anorexia, bulimia
Chronic fatigue syndrome (ME)

Culture is the way that different groups of people perceive the world and interact with their environment. It incorporates patterns of social and family relationships and religious beliefs. Cross-cultural psychiatry examines concepts of mental health and illness, their underlying causes and how symptomatology is culturally determined. It addresses issues of the universality and prevalence of psychiatric diagnoses, their treatments and their prognoses.

Concepts of symptoms, illness and healing

Our judgements concerning 'abnormal' mental symptoms or disease states frequently contain cultural assumptions of which we are unaware. For example, hallucinations and delusions of control are two of the clearest manifestations of mental illness in Western culture, but among the Xhosa of southern Africa, hallucinations confer status. More generally, 'possession states' (brief experiences of external control deliberately induced by ritual and/or drugs) are regarded as normal and indeed valued in many cultures.

Most people who have depression in any culture experience psychological and physical symptoms. In Western cultures, psychological symptoms are predominant in our concepts of psychiatric illness, while somatic symptoms are often dismissed. This 'psychologization' of depression stems from the dominance of mind/body dualism (which views the mind and body as separate) in Western countries. So while the greater likelihood of people from non-Western cultures presenting with somatic symptoms of distress has previously been labelled a peculiarity of their culture, as evidenced in many of the culture-bound syndromes described later, the difference may in fact be related more to Western cultural peculiarities.

Cultural attitudes to death and loss are particularly important in interpreting an individual's experience of bereavement. Stages of 'normal' grieving may be very different in, for example, Great Britain, India and Greece; cultural norms cannot be ignored in diagnosing 'abnormal' grief reactions. The diagnosis of personality disorder is particularly dependent on such cultural norms. For example, within Western countries, the 'dissocial' personality may be understandable and even have survival value in individuals from deprived inner-city areas with chronic exposure to violent crime, particularly where these are not offset by a stable family environment.

Culture may also influence attitudes to healing, a concept which may be wider in non-Western societies, taking into account kinship relationships and links with the supernatural world. Elaborate rituals are often involved. Acceptance of treatment implies a shared belief in illness and in the legitimacy of intervention. Some Christian sects may accept conventional diagnoses, but nonetheless oppose treatment as interference with God's will.

Culture and standardized diagnosis

Diagnostic criteria are not free from cultural influence. An extreme example of this was seen in the former Soviet Union, where the diagnosis of 'sluggish schizophrenia' was created to label political dissenters as mentally ill. The Kraepelinian approach to psychiatric diagnosis and classification (see Chapter 3), itself a reflection of Western culture and not culture-independent, remains central to ICD-10 and DSM-IV-TR. Patterns of symptoms and signs are elicited in order to make a diagnosis. The 'reliability' (or reproducibility) of such symptoms and signs across cultures is, however, questionable. The World Health Organization carried out a cross-cultural investigation of the process of psychiatric diagnosis, the International Pilot Study on Schizophrenia (IPSS), in the 1960s and 1970s. The IPSS showed that, although psychotic symptoms (delusions and hallucinations) elicited from individual patient interviews showed satisfactory reliability, clinical signs (e.g. incongruous or flat affect) were much less reliable, and corroborative evidence (e.g. from family, work and social background) less so still. At diagnostic level, psychotic disorders (including psychotic depression and schizophrenia) could be identified reliably, but neurotic (anxiety/depression) and dissociative diagnoses were much less secure. Many so-called 'culture-bound' syndromes have dissociative features.

As a step towards the recognition of these issues, DSM-IV-TR (although retaining multiple cultural assumptions within the axes of 'psychosocial and environmental problems' and 'global functioning') contains an 'outline' for 'cultural formulation'.

Culture and epidemiology

The IPSS established that the prevalence of schizophrenia was remarkably stable across cultures, although its prognosis was better in non-Western societies. This may reflect greater availability of home support without high expressed emotion and the absence of a stigmatizing label of chronic schizophrenia. In contrast, the prevalence of depression was much more variable, and its presentation in non-Western groups was often with somatic symptoms. Even for schizophrenia, cultural factors within a multicultural society may influence prevalence. For example, in the UK an excess prevalence of schizophrenia is reported among African-Caribbeans, and Irish people have particularly high rates of psychiatric hospital admissions. In both cases, higher rates of socioeco-

nomic disadvantage in these groups, a greater likelihood of experiencing disadvantage and racism or the complex interaction between immigration and mental illness are possible explanations. The excess of schizophrenia in African-Caribbean people is highest in the second generation; there is no clear consensus about why this is, although in addition to the issues discussed above, misdiagnosis of affective disorders or cultural expressions of distress as schizophrenia; and differential responses by police, social and treatment services to Black people compared with other ethnic groups have been suggested.

Another area of concern is the high rate of overdosing among South Asian women compared to White British women, which might reflect 'culture conflict' in this group. Older African-Caribbean people in the UK appear to be at greater risk of vascular dementia due to their higher prevalence of hypertension and other cardiovascular risk factors.

Pharmacological response across cultures

Racial differences in distribution of enzyme polymorphisms are reflected in, for example, increased sensitivity to alcohol (and decreased prevalence of alcohol dependence) in people of Asian origin, who also appear more susceptible to drug-induced dyskinesias. Similarly, Black Americans tend to develop higher plasma levels for given doses of tricyclic antidepressants and lithium than their White counterparts, with resultant increased sensitivity to both therapeutic and adverse affects.

Culture-bound syndromes

These denote patterns of symptoms or abnormal behaviour that are only recognized as illnesses in specific cultures. DSM-IV describes several such syndromes. ICD-10, however, does not, so in this diagnostic system they would be coded according to the symptoms experienced (e.g. under dissociative or somatoform disorders; see Chapter 27). Many have been described, mostly representing somatic and/or dissociative responses to stress. A few of the better known are outlined below.

Amok, described in Africa, Asia and New Guinea, is a response to humiliation involving initial brooding, followed by a period of altered consciousness with uncontrollable (usually homicidal and sometimes suicidal) rage, for which the subject has no subsequent memory. Traditionally, surviving sufferers were immune from legal redress, much as the French *crime passionnel*.

Ataque de nervios occurs in Hispanic American groups, and consists of a grief reaction characterized by fluctuating conscious level (often with subsequent amnesia), crying, shouting, trembling and difficulty in moving limbs. Hyperventilation may be important in precipitating symptoms.

Latah, which occurs in Asia and North Africa, is a response to intense stress characterized by altered consciousness, hypersuggestibility and mimicry (including echolalia and echopraxia).

Koro, found mainly in Asia, involves intense anxiety centred on the belief that the genitalia are retracting and that their disappearance will result in death. The traditional management is to tie a string around the penis and pull. *Koro* is associated with local tradition that ghosts have no genitals and is thus not delusional.

Brain fag is found mainly in African students, and is characterized by concentration difficulties, vague somatic complaints and depressed mood.

Some 'Western' syndromes, including multiple personality disorder, overdosing, anorexia nervosa, bulimia nervosa and chronic fatigue syndrome, may also be considered culture-bound.

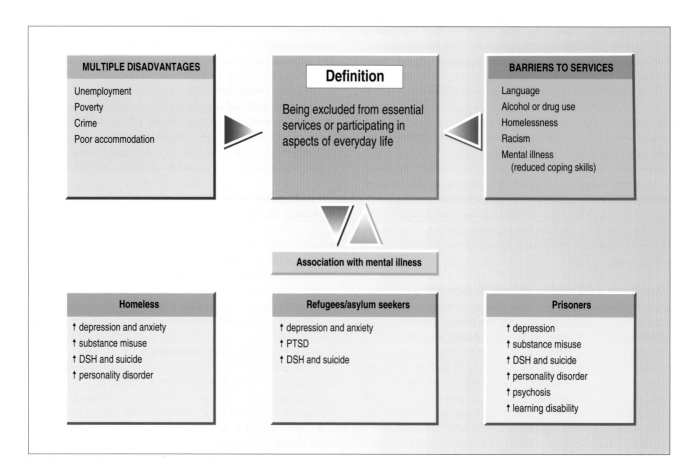

Social exclusion describes the experience of being prevented from accessing essential services or participating in everyday life. It usually results from multiple disadvantages and perhaps an inability to negotiate meeting complex needs arising from those disadvantages. Those who are socially excluded can become trapped in a cycle of unemployment, poverty, crime, poor quality accommodation or homelessness. Mental illness may be the cause or result of social exclusion.

In this chapter we look at the mental health of homeless people, immigrants/asylum seekers and prisoners. We also discuss how mental health services have tried to reduce the barriers these groups are likely to experience accessing help for psychiatric disorders. In all three groups, people's socio-economic status and experiences vary as much as in the general population. For example, asylum seekers are defined legally, not on their plight, experience of asylum or status or income in their home country. The likelihood of experiencing a severe mental illness varies with gender (commoner in women), ethnicity (see Chapter 23) and degree of economic disadvantage in these groups as in the general population.

Homeless people

A minority of homeless people are rough sleepers; many more sleep in squats, on friends' floors, in night shelters or in temporary accommodation. The stress of being homeless can lead to mental health problems. In addition, people with mental illness often find it more difficult to find accommodation and sustain a tenancy, through, for example, timely payment of bills. It is therefore sometimes difficult to discern which came first, the homelessness or the mental illness. Those with drug and alcohol problems may also find themselves excluded from accommodation. Hostels are often the only other option for people who are street homeless. A hostel can be a chaotic, frightening environment, as many residents have a long history of drug and alcohol misuse, as well as antisocial behaviour. This results in many people, especially those who are vulnerable and have mental illness, opting to sleep rough.

Around 35% of homeless people sleeping in hostels or short-term accommodation have a mental illness; this is $2^1/_2$ times the rate in the general population. Among those who are rough sleepers, rates may be as high as 60%. The prevalence of alcohol dependence and illicit drug use is also increased; an estimated 70% of rough sleepers are dependent on alcohol and 50% use illicit drugs. Personality disorders are common among the homeless.

Only 58% of rough sleepers are registered with a GP, so accessing treatment for physical and mental health may be difficult. The average life expectancy for male and female rough sleepers in central London was reported by Grenier in a 1996 study as 42 years, compared with 74 and 79 years for men and women respectively in the general population. For many homeless people with mental illness, the intricacies of primary care, including booked appointments and the low tolerance of staff and the general population to their presence, can be a significant barrier.

Many homeless people have a past history of impoverished childhood with an absence of a caring environment. This may cause difficulties forming relationships in adulthood, including the relationships with health professionals required to access help. In many areas, dedicated teams provide psychiatric and medical care for homeless people, in hostels, day centres, outpatient centres and, where necessary, the street. This more targeted, flexible outreach service can reach a far higher number of homeless people and provide care which they find acceptable. It is however, more expensive.

Asylum seekers and refugees

Nearly 1% of the world's population are refugees or displaced people. In addition to the traumas from which they are fleeing (including torture, bereavement and political repression), refugees may lose their social network, profession and financial means when they leave their homes. They often take extreme, sometimes fatal, risks to travel to their destination country. They arrive in a country where the language and culture may be unfamiliar, and may face racism and serious economic hardship. Fewer than 10% of refugees living in Western countries, including children, meet the criteria for post-traumatic stress disorder (PTSD) according to best available evidence.

Asylum-seekers (those waiting for the government to decide if they will be granted refugee status) may face a particularly anxious time and uncertain future. Some are held in detention centres on arrival, or 'dispersed' to areas of the country some distance from their point of arrival. Access to welfare and housing is restricted and they cannot legally work. Forced unemployment among asylum seekers can lead to disability from which they cannot recover, as employment permits income and a positive role in society that can mitigate the mental health consequences of seeking asylum in a society where they may be seen as competitors for resources.

Most applications for asylum are rejected, and those who remain in the country after their application has been refused may be particularly vulnerable, as they lose access to all benefits, accommodation, health and social care (except emergency care) and face deportation to the country from which they fled. They may also experience considerable difficulty in accessing primary and (particularly) secondary healthcare. Asylum seekers probably experience higher rates of anxiety, depression and PTSD than the general population, and high rates of suicide have been reported among those whose application have been refused or who are held in detention. Treatment of mental illness in asylum seekers may be complicated by homelessness and drug misuse, as well as by bereavement and lack of social support.

Asylum seekers and refugees may face difficulties in accessing psychiatric treatment, including language barriers (underlining the importance of using interpreters where needed) and lack of information about how to access local services. One study reported that 11% of patients in an inner London community mental health team were asylum seekers,

and the most frequent diagnoses in this group were depression and PTSD. They were accessing few health and social services despite having a high level of need.

Prisoners

In a recent large survey in Britain, half of men and two-thirds of women in prison reported experiencing clinically significant depression or anxiety in the preceding week. A quarter of female prisoners and one in eight male prisoners attempted suicide in the year before entering prison, and 5–10% had harmed themselves while in prison. Rates of psychosis are also higher than in the general population, with 14% of female and 8% of male prisoners experiencing a psychotic illness in the last year.

There are a number of reasons for this high prevalence of mental illness. People in prison are more likely to have experienced social adversity (unstable housing, no qualifications, unemployment) before entering prison. Being in prison is usually stressful; many prisoners have few people to confide in and physical or sexual violence is fairly common. People who have more social support, fewer recent stressful life-events and who were working and married before entering prison are more likely to remain mentally healthy while in prison, but the proportion of such people in the prison system is low.

Two-thirds of male prisoners and half of female prisoners have a personality disorder, most frequently antisocial, paranoid or, in female prisoners, borderline personality disorder. Half the prison population have an IQ of ≤85. Over 40% report dependence on drugs in the year before prison, and despite serious attempts by the prison service to keep illicit substances out of prisons, over a third report using drugs during their prison term. Drug use is particularly high among people charged with burglary, robbery and theft, suggesting that the high costs of illicit drugs may be a factor in their criminality.

In the past most psychiatric care in prison was provided by prison doctors, who referred to local psychiatric services when required. In response to concerns that prisoners were receiving a low standard of care compared with the general population, Community Mental Health In-Reach Teams have been set up in many prisons. People who have committed serious offences (murder, rape or serious violent offences) usually receive the psychiatric care required from regional forensic services.

Prisoners who are seriously mentally ill cannot be compulsorily treated within the prison system, since the Mental Health Act does not recognize prison hospital wings as hospitals within the meaning of the Act. These prisoners must be transferred to psychiatric units (usually secure units) with the agreement of the courts. High secure psychiatric facilities such as Broadmoor, Rampton and Ashworth are classified as hospitals, although they are run in close partnership with the prison system.

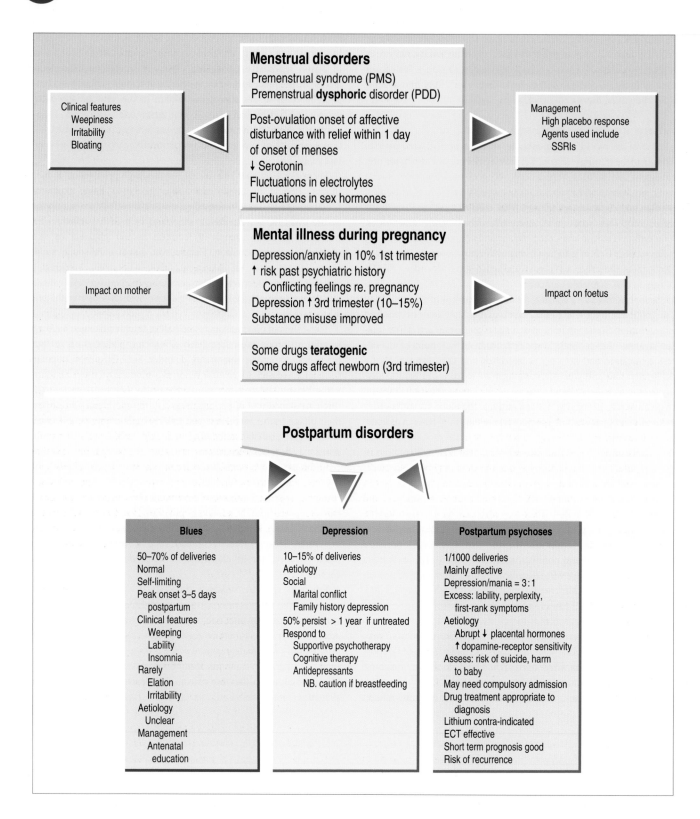

Menstrual disorders

Premenstrual syndrome (PMS)
Premenstrual **dysphoric** disorder (PDD)

Post-ovulation onset of affective
disturbance with relief within 1 day
of onset of menses
↓ Serotonin
Fluctuations in electrolytes
Fluctuations in sex hormones

Clinical features
  Weepiness
  Irritability
  Bloating

Management
  High placebo response
  Agents used include
    SSRIs

Mental illness during pregnancy

Depression/anxiety in 10% 1st trimester
↑ risk past psychiatric history
   Conflicting feelings re. pregnancy
Depression ↑ 3rd trimester (10–15%)
Substance misuse improved

Some drugs **teratogenic**
Some drugs affect newborn (3rd trimester)

Impact on mother

Impact on foetus

Postpartum disorders

Blues	Depression	Postpartum psychoses

50–70% of deliveries
Normal
Self-limiting
Peak onset 3–5 days
  postpartum
Clinical features
  Weeping
  Lability
  Insomnia
Rarely
  Elation
  Irritability
Aetiology
  Unclear
Management
  Antenatal
   education
	10–15% of deliveries
	Aetiology
	Social
	  Marital conflict
	  Family history depression
	50% persist > 1 year if untreated
	Respond to
	  Supportive psychotherapy
	  Cognitive therapy
	  Antidepressants
	    NB. caution if breastfeeding
		1/1000 deliveries
		Mainly affective
		Depression/mania = 3:1
		Excess: lability, perplexity,
		  first-rank symptoms
		Aetiology
		  Abrupt ↓ placental hormones
		  ↑ dopamine-receptor sensitivity
		Assess: risk of suicide, harm
		  to baby
		May need compulsory admission
		Drug treatment appropriate to
		  diagnosis
		Lithium contra-indicated
		ECT effective
		Short term prognosis good
		Risk of recurrence

The premenstrual syndrome (PMS)

PMS represents a disturbance of mood, often accompanied by insomnia, poor concentration, irritability, poor impulse control, food craving and physical complaints (headache, breast tenderness and bloating). The onset is after ovulation, with rapid relief within 24 hours of the onset of menstrual flow. In DSM-IV-TR it is categorized as Premenstrual Dysphoric Disorder (PDD); in ICD-10 it is listed as a physical disorder. Up to 95% of women of reproductive age have some premenstrual symptoms, but only 3–8% meet the criteria for PDD. Possible aetiological factors include a decrease in serotonin levels after ovulation, fluctuations in electrolyte and sex hormone levels and consequent neurotransmitter changes. Selective serotonin reuptake inhibitors (SSRIs) have proved beneficial. High placebo response rates have been reported in studies of PMS.

Mental illness during pregnancy

Significant depression or anxiety occurs in about 10% of women in the first trimester. Those with a past psychiatric history or with conflicting feelings about the pregnancy (such as a past or currently contemplated termination) are at particular risk. Recent evidence suggests that depression may also be common in the third trimester (10–15%). The risk of psychosis is increased postpartum, though this is not the case during pregnancy. Pregnancy often has a beneficial effect on alcohol and drug misuse. Some drugs are teratogenic (e.g. alcohol, LSD and possibly cocaine) or associated with intrauterine growth retardation or withdrawal in the newborn (e.g. opiates, alcohol). There is some evidence that the rate of suicide and suicide attempts may be reduced in pregnancy; where suicide attempts do occur, these are often associated with substance misuse.

A number of psychiatric drugs are known to have adverse effects on the foetus or newborn. Some (e.g. lithium, carbamazepine, sodium valproate, neuroleptics) increase the risk of congenital malformations. Others can affect the newborn if given in the third trimester (e.g. antipsychotics can induce an extrapyramidal syndrome, anxiolytics can cause 'floppy baby syndrome', SSRIs are associated with a neonatal behavioural syndrome, and paroxetine with pulmonary hypertension). Potential benefits of prescribing in individual cases must be weighed against these risks. Antidepressants and antipsychotics are prescribed safely in many pregnancies; long-established drugs for which there is more evidence regarding safety in pregnancy are preferred.

Postpartum disorders

These range from the mild, common and transient postpartum blues, to postpartum depression and psychoses. Risk of postpartum disorders appears similar after perinatal death (and less after abortion) to that after normal pregnancy and childbirth. Adequate opportunity to grieve should be provided, and bereavement counselling may be required. Formal psychiatric illness following termination of pregnancy is rare, but guilt feelings are common, need ventilating and may re-emerge in subsequent pregnancies. Women who have a history of serious mental illness, postpartum or otherwise, have a risk of recurrence after childbirth of 1 in 2–3. There is an increased risk of relapse after childbirth in affective disorders and probably also schizophrenia. It is important to ask about psychiatric history at the antenatal clinic so that anticipatory management plans can be made.

Postpartum blues

Postpartum blues occur after 50–70% of deliveries and should not be regarded as abnormal. The cardinal features are affective, with marked emotional lability, crying without external cause, irritability, sleep disturbance and disproportionate fear of inability to cope with the baby. Onset may be at any time within the first 10 postpartum days but is typically on days 3–5. More rarely, the blues may present (usually on day 1 or 2) with elation and irritability. The aetiology remains unclear; women with a history of severe PMS are at higher risk; elevated antepartum progesterone levels and precipitate postpartum falls in oestrogen, progesterone and sodium have been implicated. The blues are self-limiting, usually within a few days. No specific intervention is required (apart from reassurance), although more persistent depression must be excluded. Appropriate antenatal education to warn expectant mothers and their partners about the blues is helpful.

Postpartum depression

Postpartum depression occurs in 10–15% of new mothers, with onset within the first six weeks after delivery. Clinical features are similar to those of depression at other times, though suicidal thoughts are less common and guilt concerning the baby common. Unlike the blues, postpartum depression persists for a year or more in 25% of cases. Many cases of depression are undetected, either prior to or following birth, and screening for depression is an appropriate part of the six-week postnatal check. Aetiological factors appear to be predominantly social (although a family history of depression, particularly postpartum, is common), with marital conflicts and a lack of confiding relationships particularly implicated. Management involves full psychosocial assessment (including possible risk to the baby), and treatment may include marital therapy, individual (supportive or cognitive) psychotherapy and/or antidepressants. Most antidepressants are excreted in breast milk in concentrations approximating those in maternal plasma. Risks to breast-fed babies are slight, but must be considered when initiating antidepressants in women keen to continue breastfeeding. Although deliberate self-harm and suicide are less common in pregnancy and the postpartum year than at other times, suicide is still the principal cause of maternal death in the UK and may be particularly associated with death of the infant in the first year. Interruption to the development of the normally intense emotional mother–baby bond may occur. Prolonged maternal depression may also affect later social and cognitive development of the child, particularly boys, even after resolution of the maternal illness.

Postpartum psychoses

Postpartum psychoses occur after about one birth in 1000, and usually have an abrupt onset within 2–4 weeks after delivery. The clinical presentation is usually affective, the majority depressive but up to one-third with mania. Postpartum onset of schizophrenia is relatively rare, but postpartum affective psychoses are often associated with one or more Schneiderian first-rank symptoms, and are likely to show emotional lability and to be subjectively confused. Assessment of suicide risk and of risk to the baby (who may suffer from neglect, inappropriate care, deliberate harm or even infanticide) is essential. Treatment usually requires hospitalization, sometimes compulsorily and, where possible, with the baby to a specialist mother-and-baby unit. Drug treatment is as appropriate to the clinical presentation, although specialist advice is appropriate (lithium is contraindicated) in breastfeeding mothers. Electroconvulsive therapy (ECT) has been reported to be particularly effective, irrespective of diagnostic group. Short-term prognosis is excellent. Risk of postpartum recurrence is at least 1 in 3 after one postpartum episode, and up to 1 in 2 after multiple episodes. Risk appears highest in primiparae, and after instrumental delivery.

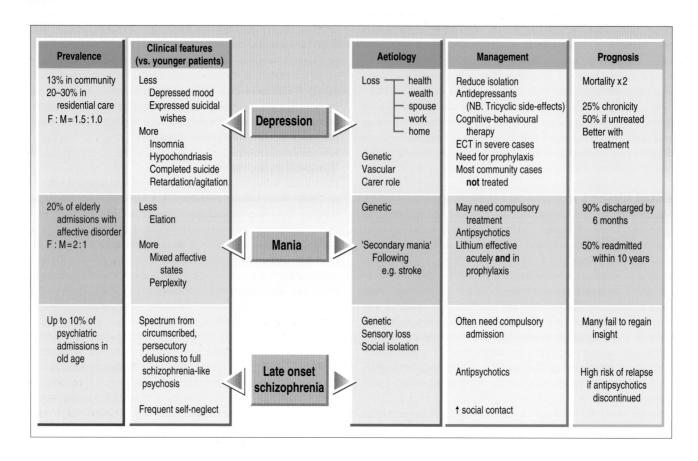

Prevalence	Clinical features (vs. younger patients)		Aetiology	Management	Prognosis

13% in community 20–30% in residential care F : M = 1.5 : 1.0	Less
	  Depressed mood
	  Expressed suicidal
	    wishes
	More
	  Insomnia
	  Hypochondriasis
	  Completed suicide
	  Retardation/agitation
		Depression	Loss ── health
			     ── wealth
			     ── spouse
			     ── work
			     ── home
			
			Genetic
			Vascular
			Carer role
				Reduce isolation
				Antidepressants
				  (NB. Tricyclic side-effects)
				Cognitive-behavioural
				  therapy
				ECT in severe cases
				Need for prophylaxis
				Most community cases
				  not treated
					Mortality x 2
					
					25% chronicity
					50% if untreated
					Better with
					  treatment

20% of elderly admissions with affective disorder F : M = 2 : 1	Less
	  Elation
	
	More
	  Mixed affective
	    states
	  Perplexity
		Mania	Genetic
			
			'Secondary mania'
			Following
			  e.g. stroke
				May need compulsory
				  treatment
				Antipsychotics
				Lithium effective
				  acutely **and** in
				  prophylaxis
					90% discharged by
					  6 months
					
					50% readmitted
					  within 10 years

Up to 10% of psychiatric admissions in old age	Spectrum from circumscribed, persecutory delusions to full schizophrenia-like psychosis
	
	Frequent self-neglect
		Late onset schizophrenia	Genetic
			Sensory loss
			Social isolation
				Often need compulsory
				  admission
				
				Antipsychotics
				
				↑ social contact
					Many fail to regain
					  insight
					
					High risk of relapse
					  if antipsychotics
					  discontinued

Older people suffer from a range of functional psychiatric disorders which may present particular problems in both detection and treatment. The most important of these (depression, mania and the delusional [schizophrenia-like] disorders of late life) are discussed below. Older people are also liable to experience adjustment reactions (particularly bereavement), although the presentation and management of these are essentially the same as earlier in life. In addition, anxiety disorders (both generalized and phobic) are common. General anxiety is often relatively mild or coexistent with (and responsive to the same treatment approaches as) depression. New episodes of phobic disorder, particularly agoraphobia, are often precipitated by traumatic events and frequently persist. Finally, older people may continue to manifest disorders of personality, although the degree of distress and disability they cause often decreases with age.

Depression in old age
Epidemiology and clinical features
Depression is about as common in late as in middle life. It affects around 13% of older people. Most studies find an over-representation of women (by a factor of about 1.5). Increased age does not automatically lead to depression. Associations between the prevalence of depression and age

are largely accounted for by physical morbidity and disability. The diagnosis is, however, often missed in older subjects, despite the fact that they frequently consult their GP; most subjects detected in community surveys have not been treated. This is partly because of the unjustified idea that depression is an inevitable consequence of ageing and also because of important differences in clinical presentation. Depressed mood is less often overt in older depressed subjects, who are also less likely to express suicidal ideation despite being at substantially higher actual risk of completed suicide. Older depressed subjects are, however, more likely to complain of disturbed sleep (which must be distinguished from the more insidious loss of sleep duration commonly found in normal ageing); to describe multiple physical problems for which no cause can be found and to exhibit motor disturbance (retardation and/or agitation). Due to these differences, conventional diagnostic criteria for depression can be misleading in old age, since the majority of subjects fulfil criteria for only 'minor' depression despite similar severity of illness to those with major depression.

Aetiology
Genetic factors are significant, although the family history is less often positive than in younger depressed patients. People who become

depressed for the first time in late life often have a low genetic loading, but are more likely to have brain-imaging abnormalities and poor treatment response. This suggests that late first-onset depression may, in some cases, reflect neurodegenerative change. This is supported by a well-documented association between vascular risk factors and depression in later life; about 20% of people with coronary artery disease develop depression. Older people with *vascular depression* may be at increased risk of developing dementia; conversely, dementia is a risk factor for developing depression. Social isolation, particularly the lack of confiding relationships, renders older people vulnerable to depression, which is often triggered by the experience of loss(es), such as bereavement, deteriorating physical health or financial insecurity. Risk of depression is also high in carers of people with dementia. Being in residential or nursing care doubles the risk of depression in old age.

Management

Both physical and psychological treatments are effective, but are under-used in older subjects. Reducing social isolation may also be important (through, for example, hearing aids and glasses, and day centre referral). Cognitive behavioural therapy may need to be modified to the needs of an older group but is effective in group as well as individual settings. Development in the last 20 years of antidepressants with a relative lack of contraindications and favourable side-effect profiles (e.g. selective serotonin reuptake inhibitors [SSRIs], venlafaxine, mirtazapine) have been critical for the effective treatment of depression in older people, though randomized placebo-controlled trial evidence for efficacy is limited. Tricyclic antidepressants are effective but usually avoided due to the higher risk of clinically important side-effects, particularly postural hypotension and resultant falls. Adherence to antidepressant treatment may be difficult to achieve in older subjects, particularly since they may take longer (up to eight weeks) to take effect. However, if there is little or no response to an adequate antidepressant at four weeks a switch to an antidepressant from a different class should be considered. Electroconvulsive therapy (ECT) is very effective in more severe depression, particularly in retarded and/or deluded patients and those refusing food or fluid, in whom the risk of irreversible physical deterioration is high. Monoamine oxidase inhibitors (MAOIs) and lithium augmentation are effective in some older patients with refractory depression.

Prognosis

Depression in late life carries a mortality rate twice that in matched control subjects. Some of the excess is related to suicide, the risk of which is particularly high in older depressed men, but most is attributable to general medical morbidity. Many factors may explain this, for example, hypercortisolaemia occurs in chronic depression, patients may avoid exercise, not take medication, etc. There is also a high risk of chronicity (about 50% if untreated) and of relapse. The prognosis is considerably improved by early intervention, as longer duration of depressive episode predicts poor outcome. Secondary prevention (continuing antidepressant therapy to prevent relapse) is highly effective.

Mania in old age

Mania accounts for about 20% of all psychiatric admissions for affective disorders in older subjects. Most have a past history of depression; in about 20% the mania is precipitated by acute physical illness such as stroke. Overt elation is less often present than in mania in earlier life, although the patient generally has grandiose ideation, and the clinical picture is more usually of irritability, lability of mood and perplexity, much like that of delirium (see Chapter 31), which is thus the most important differential diagnosis. Antipsychotics are effective in acute treatment, and some (e.g. olanzapine) are affective at preventing relapse, but atypical antipsychotics must be used with particular caution in people with dementia due to increased risks of stroke (see Chapter 34). Lithium may be used both acutely and in prophylaxis, although as many as 25% of older subjects (particularly those with Parkinson's disease or dementia) develop neurotoxicity. Both therapeutic and toxic effects of lithium may occur at lower blood levels in old age; close monitoring is therefore necessary. The prognosis with treatment is good, although recurrence occurs in up to 50% by 10 years.

Psychotic disorders

Older people with psychosis may have illnesses that have continued from earlier in life or be presenting with a first episode. Symptoms are as for younger adults (see Chapter 6). Acute confusional states, delusional depression and early dementia must all be considered in the differential diagnosis. ICD-10 and DSM-IV do not distinguish between illnesses with onset in early and later life, so the diagnostic criteria for schizophrenia and other psychotic disorders (see Chapter 6) apply. However, the term paraphrenia is still in common use for psychosis with onset in later life. Recently, consensus has been reached that late onset schizophrenia refers to a disorder with onset between the ages 40 and 60, with very late onset schizophrenia occurring at age 60+.

Aetiological factors include a genetic component (with excess family history of psychiatric illness as a whole and particularly schizophrenia), sensory deprivation (particularly deafness) and longstanding social isolation. Brain-imaging abnormalities have been reported. Treatment is often difficult because of lack of insight, but response to antipsychotics, combined if possible with social reintegration, is usually good. As older people are at particular risk of tardive dyskinesia, atypical antipsychotics may be better tolerated (but see risks above). A substantial minority of patients never regain insight despite good functional recovery. Relapse is frequent if antipsychotics are withdrawn; this must be weighed up against the risk of tardive dyskinesia with their continued use.

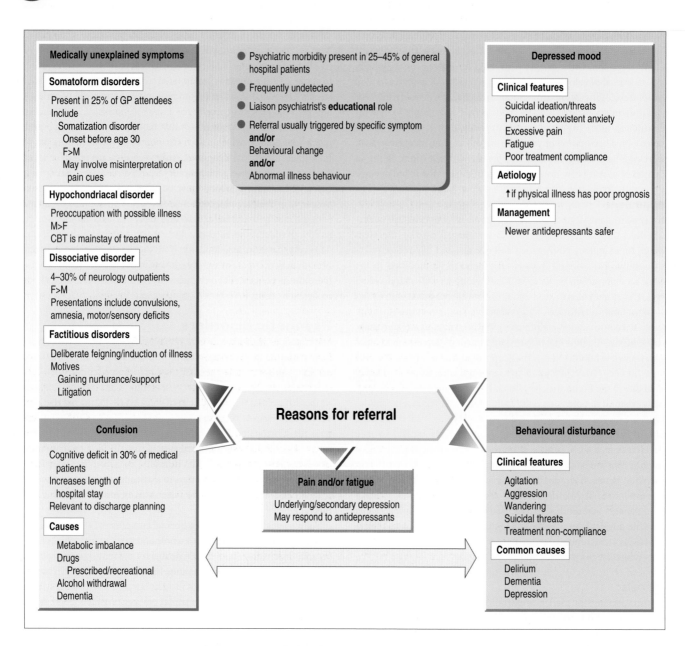

Medically unexplained symptoms

Somatoform disorders

Present in 25% of GP attendees
Include
    Somatization disorder
        Onset before age 30
        F>M
        May involve misinterpretation of
            pain cues

Hypochondriacal disorder

Preoccupation with possible illness
M>F
CBT is mainstay of treatment

Dissociative disorder

4–30% of neurology outpatients
F>M
Presentations include convulsions,
amnesia, motor/sensory deficits

Factitious disorders

Deliberate feigning/induction of illness
Motives
    Gaining nurturance/support
    Litigation

- Psychiatric morbidity present in 25–45% of general hospital patients
- Frequently undetected
- Liaison psychiatrist's **educational** role
- Referral usually triggered by specific symptom **and/or** Behavioural change **and/or** Abnormal illness behaviour

Depressed mood

Clinical features

Suicidal ideation/threats
Prominent coexistent anxiety
Excessive pain
Fatigue
Poor treatment compliance

Aetiology

↑ if physical illness has poor prognosis

Management

Newer antidepressants safer

Reasons for referral

Confusion

Cognitive deficit in 30% of medical
    patients
Increases length of
    hospital stay
Relevant to discharge planning

Causes

Metabolic imbalance
Drugs
    Prescribed/recreational
Alcohol withdrawal
Dementia

Pain and/or fatigue

Underlying/secondary depression
May respond to antidepressants

Behavioural disturbance

Clinical features

Agitation
Aggression
Wandering
Suicidal threats
Treatment non-compliance

Common causes

Delirium
Dementia
Depression

Comorbidity of psychiatric and physical illness

Psychiatric morbidity (consisting mainly of organic disorders, depression and anxiety) is present in a high (25–45%) proportion of medical and surgical patients, largely irrespective of their primary diagnosis. This reflects psychiatric disturbances secondary to physical illness, side-effects from medications and the increased physical vulnerability that psychiatric difficulties impart. As many as 30% of acute medical patients have some cognitive deficits, reflecting in part the vulnerability of older people to both cognitive and physical disorders. Delirium (see Chapter 31), depression and anxiety disorders are much commoner among those with physical illnesses. In addition, certain personality traits may predispose to specific physical illness; for example, aggressiveness, hostility and competitive striving ('type A' behaviours) may

predispose to myocardial infarction. Dementia (see Chapter 32) may first become apparent in the setting of acute physical illness, as patients reveal their inability to learn to cope in a novel environment and without family support. Dementia is associated with increased length of hospital stay and its early detection may facilitate appropriate discharge planning.

Depressed mood, anxiety symptoms and adjustment disorders (see Chapter 10) may be evident where the concurrent physical illness has a poor prognosis in terms of chronicity (e.g. diabetes), level of incapacitation or life expectancy. Supportive psychotherapy may be helpful in coming to terms with the consequences of illness. Depressive symptoms may become severe and render patients suicidal and reluctant to eat or drink, thereby increasing their physical frailty or non-compliance with medication or physiotherapy. Diagnosis can be problematic, as some symptoms of serious physical illness (such as lethargy, poor sleep and reduced appetite) can be difficult to distinguish from those of depression. In these cases it can be helpful to focus on cognitive features such as anhedonia, guilt and hopelessness. Antidepressants may be beneficial. ECT is rarely used, but can be life-saving in severe or psychotic depressive illness in physically ill people, particularly where suicidal risk is high or where physical health is further threatened by poor food and fluid intake. Structural brain disease or injury can also cause organic psychiatric disorders such as mood disorders or psychosis, the best-known example being the link between stroke (particularly following left anterior infarcts) and depression (Chapter 28).

Patients with *pre-existing psychiatric illness* may require urgent medical or surgical management. This is particularly likely in the context of alcohol or substance abuse, and in patients with established depression or schizophrenia who attempt suicide which may lead to multiple injuries. Such patients will need continued psychiatric management with careful monitoring of their mental state under stressful circumstances.

Medically unexplained symptoms

Many people experience medical symptoms for which no cause is found. There are a number of possible explanations. They may relate to an undetected physical cause; they may be physical symptoms arising from a psychiatric disorder. Many people with depression will experience physical symptoms (e.g. headaches, general malaise) as a result of their illness. Unexplained medical symptoms may also be due to a somatoform, dissociative or factitious disorder. These disorders, when severe, interfere with the individual's level of psychosocial functioning resulting in marked levels of disability.

Somatoform disorders

A quarter of GP attendees have somatoform disorders. These include somatization disorder and hypochondriacal disorder.

Somatization disorder is characterized in ICD-10 by at least two years of multiple physical symptoms with no physical explanation; the patient persistently refuses to accept the advice of doctors that there is no physical explanation, and their social and family functioning is impaired as a result of the illness. Gastrointestinal and skin complaints are most common. It is much commoner in women than in men, usually starting before the age of 30, and often results in multiple operations despite the absence of organic disorder. The experience of pain is generated by the mind, not the body. It is thought that people with somatization disorder may misinterpret normal bodily sensations or relatively mild discomfort as pain. This in turn causes them worry and stress, which may exacerbate the symptoms. The patient is not consciously aware of the origin of their symptoms, no matter how clear and sometimes frustrating this might be to their families and carers.

Hypochondriacal disorder is a non-delusional preoccupation with the possibility of serious illness such as cancer, heart disease or AIDS. It is more common in men and people who have more contact with disease (e.g. health workers). *Dysmorphophobia* is related to hypochondriacal disorder. It is an excessive preoccupation with imagined or barely noticeable defects in physical appearance. For example, patients may become preoccupied by the size of their nose, believing an objectively normal nose to be ugly and deformed. CBT is the mainstay of treatment for somatoform disorders. SSRIs can be helpful for dysmorphophobia.

Dissociative disorders

The traditional psychoanalytic view suggests that in dissociative (conversion) disorders, painful memories or thoughts (or the distress associated with them) are 'cut off' from the conscious self (Freud used the term 'repressed memories') and 'converted' into more acceptable and bearable physical symptoms. Modern psychoanalytic views see conversion disorders as resulting from ineffective communication. Diagnosis requires both the presence of physical (usually neurological) symptoms in the absence of pathology and a clear relationship with stressful events or disturbed relationships. Although rare in the general population, dissociative disorders affect between 4% and 30% of neurology outpatients; they are more common in women. Diagnoses include dissociative motor and sensory deficits, dissociative amnesia (usually upsetting and personal information is forgotten); dissociative fugue (where dissociative amnesia is associated with a seemingly purposeful unplanned journey away from home); dissociative convulsions (pseudoseizures) and Ganser's syndrome (see Chapter 16).

Management of these conditions involves ensuring that there really is no organic basis, treating any underlying mood disorder and exploring with the patient (and the family) any 'secondary gain' (such as sympathy or avoidance of family conflict) which might be encouraging symptom maintenance.

Managing pain and fatigue

Pain may trigger psychiatric referral even without clear evidence of somatoform disorder. Depression may underlie such pain or result from it, particularly if pain is inadequately treated for fear of causing opiate dependence. Chronic pain may respond to antidepressants even in the absence of clear-cut depression, and often at doses too low to be antidepressant. Similar considerations apply to fatigue, a feature common to many physical and psychiatric illnesses. In particular, the combination of exhaustion after minimal physical activity, poor concentration and muscle tenderness which constitutes Myalgic Encephalomyelitis (ME; chronic fatigue syndrome) shares many features with depression and may respond to antidepressants.

Factitious disorder

People with factitious disorder deliberately feign or actually induce illness in themselves, typically to gain the nurture of others or with a litigious aim. Munchausen's syndrome and Munchausen's syndrome by proxy (feigning illness in oneself or a dependant) fall in this category (see Chapter 16).

Liaison psychiatry

The considerable overlap of psychiatric and physical symptoms clearly necessitates close cooperation between psychiatric and medical doctors if patients are to be treated effectively. In medical and surgical wards and clinics, this is managed through the liaison psychiatry team. Patients presenting with behavioural disturbance frequently have delirium (which must be excluded, or its underlying cause identified and treated as a matter of urgency) or dementia. Suicidal threats or gestures may also cause considerable anxiety in ward nursing staff, who may need advice on assessment and management of suicide risk (see Chapter 5). Multidisciplinary discussion of behavioural problems can often identify triggers to undesirable behaviour and help ward staff find ways of defusing provocative situations.

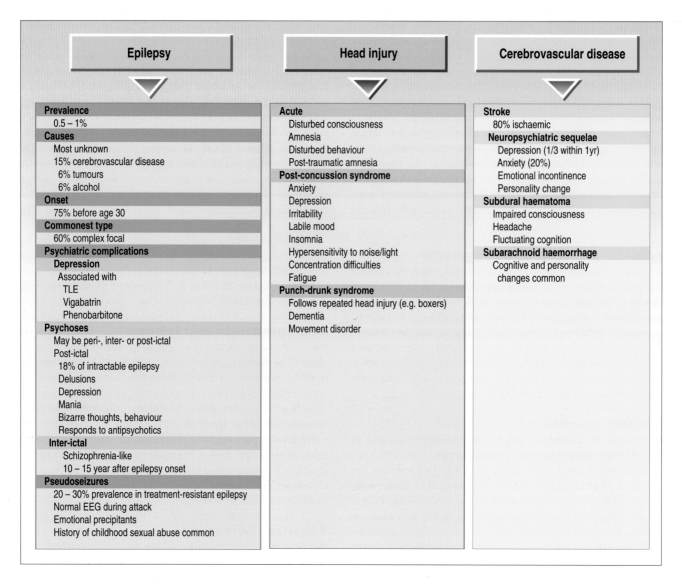

Epilepsy

Prevalence
0.5 – 1%
Causes
Most unknown
15% cerebrovascular disease
6% tumours
6% alcohol
Onset
75% before age 30
Commonest type
60% complex focal
Psychiatric complications
Depression
Associated with
TLE
Vigabatrin
Phenobarbitone
Psychoses
May be peri-, inter- or post-ictal
Post-ictal
18% of intractable epilepsy
Delusions
Depression
Mania
Bizarre thoughts, behaviour
Responds to antipsychotics
Inter-ictal
Schizophrenia-like
10 – 15 year after epilepsy onset
Pseudoseizures
20 – 30% prevalence in treatment-resistant epilepsy
Normal EEG during attack
Emotional precipitants
History of childhood sexual abuse common

Head injury

Acute
Disturbed consciousness
Amnesia
Disturbed behaviour
Post-traumatic amnesia
Post-concussion syndrome
Anxiety
Depression
Irritability
Labile mood
Insomnia
Hypersensitivity to noise/light
Concentration difficulties
Fatigue
Punch-drunk syndrome
Follows repeated head injury (e.g. boxers)
Dementia
Movement disorder

Cerebrovascular disease

Stroke
80% ischaemic
Neuropsychiatric sequelae
Depression (1/3 within 1yr)
Anxiety (20%)
Emotional incontinence
Personality change
Subdural haematoma
Impaired consciousness
Headache
Fluctuating cognition
Subarachnoid haemorrhage
Cognitive and personality
changes common

Neuropsychiatry is primarily concerned with those conditions in which mental disorder results from demonstrable structural or neurophysiological disturbance of the brain. Psychiatric aspects of organic disorders include personality and behavioural changes, cognitive difficulties, affective disturbances, psychoses and confusional states. The psychiatric picture seldom bears a specific relationship to the type of underlying pathology, being more influenced by the site of brain involvement and the time course of the illness. An organic disorder can mimic functional disorders, but features suggestive of organic problems include cognitive disorder preceding mood or other psychiatric symptoms, specific cognitive deficits suggesting focal dysfunction, neurological signs, fluctuating symptomatology, visual hallucinations, vague or transient paranoid delusions and symptoms not typical of a functional disorder. In order to make the diagnosis, full physical and neurological examinations must be undertaken, in addition to the history and mental state examination. Investigations should include a general screen (see Chapter 31). More specialized investigations may help to confirm or exclude specific diagnoses (see below). Lumbar puncture should be

undertaken with caution if raised intracranial pressure is suspected in view of the risk of precipitating brainstem coning.

In this chapter, we review the neuropsychiatric symptoms associated with epilepsy, head injury, cerebrovascular disease and tumour.

Epilepsy

The prevalence of epilepy is 0.5–1%, excluding febrile convulsions, single seizures and inactive cases. It is slightly more common in men. In most cases the cause is unknown; known causes include cerebrovascular disease (15%), cerebral tumours (6%), alcohol-related seizures (6%) and post-traumatic seizures (2%). Onset is usually before the age of 30 (75%), although the prevalence in older people is increasing as the population ages amongst whom cerebrovascular disease is greater. The commonest seizure type is complex focal (60%), 60% of which arise in the temporal lobes.

Psychiatric aspects of epilepsy may be divided into peri-ictal (relating to the ictus or seizures) and inter-ictal (disturbances are chronic and not related to the ictal electric discharge).

Depression is common in people with epilepsy; in community surveys, 20–30% of those with recurrent seizures were depressed. The commonest and clinically relevant entity is inter-ictal depression, which is more likely to be associated with agitation and psychotic features or impulsive self-harm than in people without epilepsy. Depression can directly increase seizure frequency through the mechanism of sleep deprivation.

Depression is more likely to occur in patients with temporal lobe epilepsy (TLE). Other aetiological factors include antiepileptic drugs (e.g. phenobarbitone and vigabatrin), a family history of depression, and psychosocial factors (adverse life-events, social stigmatization, financial stress, unemployment). Paradoxically, depression can follow remission of epilepsy. Suicide is increased in people with epilepsy (5 × general population; TLE 25 ×). Treatment includes careful use of antidepressants. Selective noradrenaline and serotonin uptake inhibitors (SNRIs), selective serotonin reuptake inhibitors (SSRIs) and monoamine oxidase inhibitors (MAOIs) are recommended as least likely to lower the seizure threshold. Citalopram is also least likely to interact with anti-epilepsy drugs. Electroconvulsive therapy (ECT) may be given if necessary. Carbamazepine and lamotrigine are anti-epileptic agents that may also improve mood. *Mania* and *elation* are rarely associated with epilepsy.

Psychoses related to epilepsy can occur as part of a seizure (ictal psychoses) immediately after a seizure (post-ictal psychoses), or unrelated to the timing of seizures (inter-ictal). Post-ictal psychosis may occur in up to 18% of people with intractable seizures; it should be distinguished from delirium. It occurs up to a week after the seizure and lasts from as little as a day up to three months. Symptoms may include delusions, depressive or manic psychosis or bizarre thoughts and behaviour, and usually respond well to antipsychotic medication. There is an increased incidence of 'inter-ictal' schizophrenia-like psychoses (usually paranoid) in people with epilepsy. These psychoses (which usually develop 10–15 years after the onset of epilepsy) are associated with left TLE, neurological abnormalities, negative family history of schizophrenia and a 'warm' affect, with little personality deterioration. Psychosis may occasionally follow temporal lobectomy. Treatment is with antipsychotics, preferably those with least effect on seizure threshold (e.g. sulpiride, quetiapine, haloperidol).

Cognitive impairments are common in people with epilepsy and may be caused by anti-epileptic medication (phenobarbitone, phenytoin) or persistent abnormal electrical activity in the brain between seizures. *Pseudo-seizures* simulate real seizures and occur in 20–30% of people with chronic treatment-resistant epilepsy. They are often frequent, occur when other people are present, indoors or at home, have an emotional precipitant and are associated with a history of childhood sexual abuse. Characteristically, the electroencephalogram (EEG) is normal during the attack. Most people with epilepsy have a normal personality; when a personality disorder does occur it is not of any particular kind. Sexual dysfunction is common in people with epilepsy; causes include anti-epileptic medication side-effects, neurophysiological problems (more common in TLE) and social problems.

Head injury

Both short- and long-term psychiatric disturbance may occur following head injury. Acute effects include disturbance of consciousness, amnesia and behavioural disorder. Post-traumatic amnesia describes amnesia for the injury and subsequent events and is a more accurate prognostic indicator than retrograde amnesia. Duration of loss of consciousness greater than 24 hours is associated with worse cognitive outcomes. Personality and behavioural changes may relate to the site of the injury (e.g. frontal lobe damage can result in disinhibition, aggression and impulsivity). Psychosis is commoner after temporal lobe injury. Depression occurs in up to 25%. A 'post-concussional syndrome' has been described with anxiety, depression, irritability, emotional lability, insomnia, hypersensitivity to noise/light, reduced concentration and chronic tiredness, There may be an organic basis for the syndrome, but psychological and social factors are likely to play a major role; there is no specific treatment. Repeated minor head injuries may cause 'punch drunk syndrome', where the clinical picture is of dementia with movement disorder; it classically affects retired boxers.

Cerebrovascular disease

A *cerebrovascular accident* (CVA; stroke) is a focal neurological deficit that occurs secondary to a sudden loss of blood flow to brain tissue, due to ischaemia (80%) or haemorrhage. The immediate effects of stroke depend on site; hemiparesis, sensory loss and speech disorders are common. Neuropsychiatric sequelae are frequent, particularly changes in cognition, affect (lability, depression) and personality (apathy, irritability). *Transient ischaemic attack* (TIA) describes a similar event that resolves within 24 hours.

Depression affects one third of stroke victims within one year; the aetiology is likely to involve direct neurophysiological effects as well as the psychosocial impact of sudden disability. Antidepressants are effective. Anxiety disorders (20%), apathy (20%) and emotional incontinence are also common after stroke.

Subdural haematoma results from venous bleeding into the subdural space. Presentation may be acute, but is often chronic (especially in the elderly), the causative injury having been forgotten. Features include impaired consciousness, headache and fluctuating cognition and the picture may be of dementia. *Subarachnoid haemorrhage* usually results from rupture of a cerebral artery aneurysm. Cognitive and personality changes are common in those who survive.

Progressive cerebrovascular events may result in clinical dementia (see *vascular dementia*; Chapter 32).

Tumour

Primary and secondary intracranial tumours can lead to a spectrum of behavioural, affective, psychotic, personality and cognitive disturbances via a number of mechanisms, including mass effects and obstructive hydrocephalus. Malignancy outside the cranium can also lead to neuropsychiatric disturbance as a result of tumour by-products or effects on renal, endocrine and other body systems.

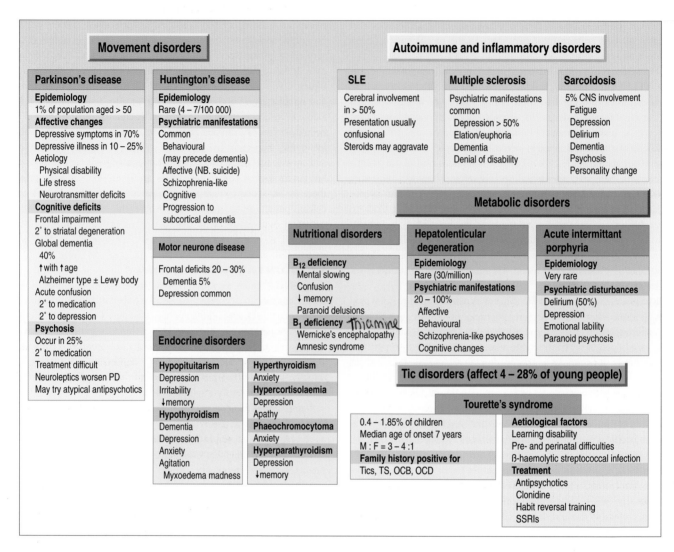

Movement disorders

Parkinson's disease (PD) affects over 1% of the population above 50 years of age and results from deficient striatal dopaminergic activity. Treatment is predominantly with anti-Parkinsonian medication. Psychiatric disturbances include intellectual impairment, affective changes and psychoses. Global dementia occurs in up to 40%; risk increases with age and duration of PD (78% after eight years). PD dementia is similar to dementia with Lewy bodies (DLB) (see Chapter 32). Coexistent Alzheimer's pathology is common. Frontal lobe cognitive deficits are seen early in PD and relate to striatal dysfunction. Isolated focal abnormalities (e.g. immediate recall of verbal material, working memory), drug-induced confusional states (especially with antimuscarinic compounds and selegiline) and depression-related cognitive difficulties are also common. Psychotic symptoms occur in 25% often in relation to their anti-PD medication; visual hallucinations and persecutory delusions are commonest. Affective disturbances may be confounded by physical symptoms of PD. Aetiology is multifactorial, involving neurotransmitter systems (dopaminergic, serotonergic, cholinergic) and psychosocial problems (low self-esteem, physical disability, poor coping strategies, dissatisfaction with support, social stress,

sexual problems). Treatment of depression and psychoses should be with drugs with a relatively low propensity to induce extrapyramidal side-effects.

Huntington's disease (HD) is characterized by cognitive decline, choreiform involuntary movements and personality change. It is inherited as an autosomal dominant gene (100% penetrance) on the short arm of chromosome 4. Rare individuals have a negative family history, which may be due to a new spontaneous mutation or mistaken parentage. HD manifests at all ages, affects men and women equally, and prevalence is 4–7/100 000. There is cerebral atrophy, and reduced γ-aminobutyric acid (GABA) resulting in dopamine hypersensitivity. Cognitive impairments usually progress to a subcortical dementia, characterized by mental slowing, impaired executive functioning and a decline in memory; speech deteriorates faster than comprehension.

Psychiatric disturbances, common in patients with HD, include changes in behaviour/personality (apathy, irritability), affective disorders (depression 40%; mania 10%) and schizophreniform psychoses. These psychiatric disorders are not related to the severity of the HD. Depression can also precede other symptoms. There is an increased risk of suicide in patients with HD and in those at risk (as high as 10%); this must be borne in mind when planning genetic counselling and predictive testing. Treatment is symptomatic, and depression and psychoses should be treated with standard medications. Death usually occurs about 15 years after diagnosis.

Motor neurone disease is a progressive neurodegenerative disease that affects the upper and lower motor neurones, leading to weakness and muscle wasting. It causes increasing loss of mobility in the limbs, and difficulties with speech, swallowing and breathing. Cognitive frontal lobe deficits occur in 20–40% of patients with MND, but only 5% have clinical dementia, usually frontotemporal (see Chapter 32). Depression is also common.

Tic disorders

Tics are very common, affecting 4–28% of young people. Possible diagnoses are transient tic disorder (tics lasting <12 months), chronic vocal or chronic motor tic disorder or *Tourette's syndrome* (TS, which requires the presence of multiple motor tics and one or more vocal tics for >12 months). Current research suggests that TS occurs in 1% of children aged 5–18 years. Males are more often affected (3–4 : 1). The family history is frequently positive for tics, TS, obsessive–compulsive behaviour (OCB) and obsessive–compulsive disorder (OCD). Both TS and tics are more common in people with learning disability and autistic spectrum disorders. Other aetiological suggestions include pre- and perinatal difficulties and some infections, particularly group A ß-haemolytic streptococcus.

TS usually begins with facial tics such as excessive blinking; the median age at onset is seven years. Tics usually improve by age 18. Associated features include attention-deficit hyperactivity disorder (ADHD) and OCB. Treatment is with antipsychotics (for tics), clonidine with or without stimulants (e.g. atomoxetine) (for ADHD), selective serotonin reuptake inhibitors (SSRIs) for depression or OCB/OCD and a behavioural approach, habit reversal training (see Chapter 33).

Autoimmune and inflammatory disorders

Multiple sclerosis (MS) is the commonest cause of neurological disability in adults of working age. It is characterized by episodes of demyelination which result in central nervous system abnormalities disseminated in time and space. Both genetic (chromosome 6 possibly responsible) and environmental factors (e.g. virus) are aetiologically important. The most frequent psychiatric complication is depression (>50% lifetime prevalence), which appears to be related to stress rather than the disease process; suicidal ideation is common. There is also an increased incidence of bipolar affective disorder. Transient psychoses and elation/euphoria may occur, often related to the disease process. Cognitive impairment (early) and progressive dementia (late) also occur. Denial of disability is common.

Systemic lupus erythematosus (SLE) is a connective tissue disorder which can present with cerebral manifestations (>50%). Characteristically, there are transient, fluctuating psychiatric disturbances of which acute confusional states (caused e.g. by CNS vasculitis, encephalopathy) are commonest. Depressive psychosis may occur less frequently. Transient psychotic phenomena may occur, although persistent schizophrenia-like psychoses are rare. Treatment with steroids may cause further psychiatric complications.

Sarcoidosis

The CNS is affected in about 5% of cases. It is associated with fatigue, depression, delirium, dementia, depression, psychosis and personality changes.

Metabolic disturbance

Hepatolenticular degeneration (also known as Wilson's disease) is an uncommon autosomal recessive disorder (chromosome 13). Psychiatric manifestations are common and may be the presenting feature in more than half of cases. The commonest psychiatric symptom clusters are affective and behavioural changes (e.g. aggression). Schizophrenia-like psychoses are relatively uncommon although cognitive changes are well recognized. Treatment is with 'anti-copper drugs' (e.g. penicillamine); psychiatric disturbances are treated with appropriate psychotropic medication.

Acute intermittent porphyria (AIP) is the commonest type of porphyria (but still very rare). Acute attacks occur spontaneously or may be precipitated by drugs (e.g. oral contraceptives, hypoglycaemics, alcohol), infections, pregnancy, metabolic and nutritional factors (e.g. low carbohydrate intake). Clinical presentation may be abdominal (colicky pain, vomiting, constipation) or neurological (peripheral neuropathy, bulbar palsies, epilepsy). Psychiatric disturbances include delirium (50%), depression, emotional lability, schizophrenia-like psychoses (especially paranoid) and symptoms incorrectly diagnosed as 'hysteria'.

Endocrine

Endocrine causes of psychiatric symptoms include pituitary, thyroid, adrenal and parathyroid abnormalities. *Hypopituitarism* (Simmond's disease) is almost invariably associated with depression, irritability and/or impaired memory.

Hypothyroidism may present as dementia, depression, anxiety or acute agitation (myxoedema madness, with features of predominantly agitated depression). *Hyperthyroidism* can be associated with anxiety, depression (which may be delusional) or occasionally apathy and loss of appetite in older people.

Hypercortisolaemia, which is most commonly iatrogenic, may induce depression or mania. *Hypocortisolaemia* (Addison's disease) is usually associated with depression and apathy. *Phaeochromocytoma* may present with episodic anxiety accompanied by labile hypertension.

Hyperparathyroidism is often accompanied by depression and apathy and occasionally by memory deficits and psychotic symptoms. *Primary hypoparathyroidism* usually presents insidiously with emotional lability, poor concentration and cognitive impairment. When it is secondary to removal of parathyroid glands, presentation may be with an acute confusional state or psychosis.

Nutritional disorders

Vitamin B_{12} deficiency results in pernicious anaemia. This may be accompanied by subacute combined degeneration of the spinal cord, which is associated with signs of neuropathy and spinal cord involvement. Psychiatric symptoms include slowing of mental processes, confusion, memory problems, intellectual impairment (all associated with low serum B_{12}), depression and paranoid delusions. Treatment is with hydroxycobalamin. *Thiamine (B_1)* deficiency can result in Wernicke's encephalopathy and the amnesic syndrome of Korsakoff's psychosis (see Chapter 18). In the developed world, this is most commonly associated with alcohol dependence. The underlying pathology is of mammillary body damage.

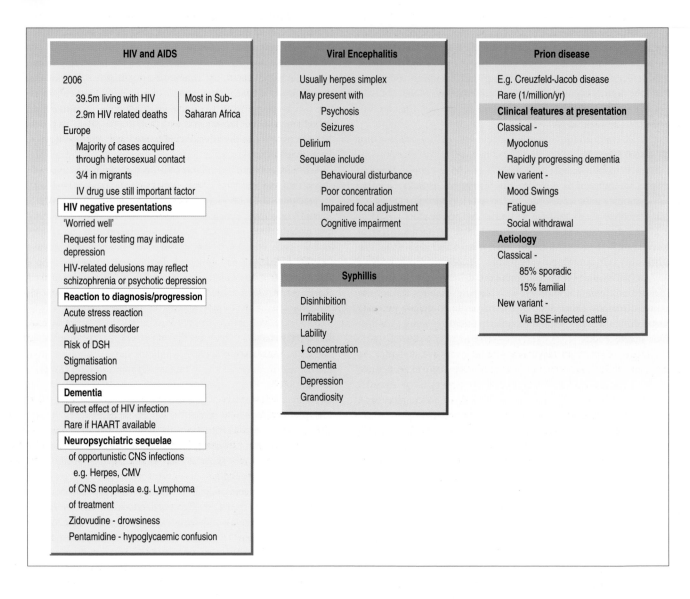

HIV and AIDS

2006

39.5m living with HIV | Most in Sub-
2.9m HIV related deaths | Saharan Africa

Europe

Majority of cases acquired through heterosexual contact

3/4 in migrants

IV drug use still important factor

HIV negative presentations

'Worried well'

Request for testing may indicate depression

HIV-related delusions may reflect schizophrenia or psychotic depression

Reaction to diagnosis/progression

Acute stress reaction

Adjustment disorder

Risk of DSH

Stigmatisation

Depression

Dementia

Direct effect of HIV infection

Rare if HAART available

Neuropsychiatric sequelae

of opportunistic CNS infections
  e.g. Herpes, CMV

of CNS neoplasia e.g. Lymphoma

of treatment

Zidovudine - drowsiness

Pentamidine - hypoglycaemic confusion

Viral Encephalitis

Usually herpes simplex

May present with
  Psychosis
  Seizures

Delirium

Sequelae include
  Behavioural disturbance
  Poor concentration
  Impaired focal adjustment
  Cognitive impairment

Syphillis

Disinhibition

Irritability

Lability

↓ concentration

Dementia

Depression

Grandiosity

Prion disease

E.g. Creuzfeld-Jacob disease

Rare (1/million/yr)

Clinical features at presentation

Classical -
  Myoclonus
  Rapidly progressing dementia

New varient -
  Mood Swings
  Fatigue
  Social withdrawal

Aetiology

Classical -
  85% sporadic
  15% familial

New variant -
  Via BSE-infected cattle

HIV and AIDS

The World Health Organization estimated that in 2006, 39.5 million people were living with human immunodeficiency virus (HIV) or acquired immunodeficiency syndrome (AIDS) and 2.9 million died of AIDS-related illnesses, of whom 2.1 million were in sub-Saharan Africa. In the developed world, the prevalence is rising, in part due to the life-prolonging effects of antiretroviral therapy. In the UK the incidence of new HIV diagnoses has trebled since 2000. In Western Europe, more than half of new diagnoses were acquired through heterosexual contact, three-quarters in migrants or immigrants. Intravenous drug abusers remain a high-risk group, despite harm-reduction strategies.

In Western countries, people with HIV who commence and adhere to an effective treatment regimen before their immune system has been severely damaged can now live a relatively normal lifespan. Earlier predictions that rising rates of infection would result in an epidemic of HIV-related dementia and other end-stage diseases have thus not been realized. Associated psychological problems range from fear of infection in the 'worried well', through psychological reactions to being HIV-infected, to functional psychiatric disorders in those with established HIV and neuropsychiatric syndromes in the minority (in the West) who develop full-blown AIDS.

The worried well

People (not all of whom are at risk of HIV) may become preoccupied with the possibility of becoming infected; this may present with repeated requests for HIV serological testing. HIV testing provides an opportunity for education on minimizing high-risk behaviour. A request for testing may reflect underlying depression or anxiety, which should be excluded or treated as part of the initial assessment. More rarely, patients with psychotic depression or schizophrenia may present with the delusion that they are HIV-positive.

Psychological reactions to HIV infection

Patients with HIV may undergo periods of crisis on first learning that they are infected, starting retroviral treatment, if tests indicate a problem with treatment (CD4 count rising or drug resistance) or when they first develop an HIV-related illness. They may react to these crises with acute stress reactions or more insidious adjustment reactions (see Chapter 10). Risk of deliberate self-harm must be considered. Self-help groups can play an important role. Despite treatment advances, HIV is still a stigmatizing diagnosis in many sections of society.

HIV and psychiatric illness

These are both associated with drug and alcohol use. Intravenous drug users are at directly increased risk of contracting HIV, while other substances that impair judgement or decrease inhibitions may also cause people to put themselves at risk. Similarly, other psychiatric conditions that involve increased impulsivity or risk-taking behaviours (e.g. borderline personality disorder, manic episode) may increase the risk of infection. There is therefore a sizeable population living with both HIV and psychiatric illness. Once infected, people with mental illness may be less likely to adhere to the complicated regimens of retroviral treatment. The patient's right to confidentiality may in rare cases need to be balanced against the need to protect others if health professionals become aware that they are putting others at risk (e.g. through unprotected sex).

Depression is common at all stages of HIV and AIDS. The diagnosis of depressive illness may be difficult. Apathy and fatigue are recognized adverse effects of retroviral therapy. Fatigue and weight loss may also be caused by declining CD4 counts and rising viral loads, so advancing HIV infection must also be considered in the differential diagnosis. AIDS-related dementia (now rare) may also present as a depression-like illness. Anhedonia, hopelessness and suicidal thinking are, however, likely to reflect true depressive illness and warrant treatment. Depression often reduces medication adherence and has been associated with an increase in CD4 count decline, so screening for it is an important part of HIV care. Depression may also potentiate the disabling effects of HIV and AIDS. *Suicide* is increased more than 20-fold in HIV-positive individuals.

HIV-positive patients may also present with *acute mania* or *schizophrenia-like psychoses*. Both illnesses may have been present before HIV diagnosis. New onset cases are often associated with MRI/CT brain abnormalities, suggesting organic pathology. *Anxiety* is also common and may respond to behavioural and/or pharmacological treatment. Organic aetiology should be excluded or treated; the principles of management of functional psychoses are not altered by comorbidity with HIV or AIDS. Caution is required whenever prescribing in HIV due to drug interactions and high sensitivity to side-effects, especially EPSEs.

Neuropsychiatric complications of HIV

Some people infected with HIV (estimates vary between 10% and 90%) develop self-limiting aseptic meningitis, which probably represents the entry of the virus into the CNS. The clinical presentation is usually of a glandular fever-like illness accompanied by neck stiffness, but there may also be a transient confusional state.

Later in the disease, HIV-positive subjects may develop persistent and progressive cognitive changes. These are thought to be a direct manifestation of HIV infection within the brain and are known as HIV-I associated dementia. This has become rare in the developed world since the introduction of highly active antiretroviral therapy (HAART).

Severely immunocompromised AIDS patients are vulnerable to a variety of opportunistic CNS infections. Viral infections include herpes and cytomegalovirus (CMV). Non-viral infections are also common and include tuberculosis (TB), syphilis, toxoplasmosis, candidiasis and cryptococcal meningitis. AIDS also renders patients vulnerable to CNS neoplasia, particularly lymphoma (primary or secondary) and metastatic Kaposi's sarcoma. CNS vasculitis can result in haemorrhage or infarction. These complications may present with non-specific cognitive deterioration or more florid acute confusional states, with or without focal neurological signs.

Treatments directed at HIV and its complications can also result in neuropsychiatric syndromes. Zidovudine can cause drowsiness or, rarely, a mania-like syndrome. Pentamidine (used in the treatment and prophylaxis of cryptococcal lung infections) may induce hypoglycaemia and resultant confusion.

Viral encephalitis

The commonest cause of viral encephalitis in the West is herpes simplex. While presentation is usually with severe headache, vomiting and reduced consciousness, patients may occasionally present with psychosis, seizures or delirium. At least 50% of survivors experience disturbances of behaviour, concentration or social adjustment, with chronic cognitive impairment in some.

Syphilis

Syphilis (*Treponema pallidum* infection) has three stages: primary (a chancre [sore] at the site of inoculation); secondary (rashes, fever, joint pains); after which about a third progress after some years (often a decade) to tertiary (rare today due to treatment with penicillin). Symptoms of tertiary syphilis can affect the brain (neurosyphilis, causing optic atrophy, tabes dorsalis and general paralysis of the insane [GPI]). Tabes dorsalis presents with lightning pains, ataxia, paraesthesias and Argyll-Robertson pupils (small, irregular, reactive to convergence but not to light). GPI may include personality (disinhibition, irritability, lability) and cognitive (poor concentration) changes, dementia (20–40%), depression (25%), grandiosity (10%) and, more rarely, mania and schizophrenia-like psychoses. Intramuscular penicillin remains the first-line treatment. The main blood test for syphilis is VDRL.

Prion disease

Human forms of *spongiform encephalopathy* (prion disorders, e.g. Creutzfeld–Jacob disease [CJD]) are rare (1/million per year) and are characterized by accumulation of an abnormal form of a normal host protease-resistant protein (PrP) in the brain. They present with a rapidly fatal dementia associated with myoclonic jerks. About 85% of cases are sporadic; the remaining cases of classical CJD are either familial (15%; sometimes autosomal dominant) or very rarely iatrogenic. A new form of CJD (variant CJD) was reported in younger adults (average age 27) in the UK in 1996 and appeared to relate to consumption of beef from cattle affected by bovine spongiform encephalopathy (BSE). Whereas classic CJD usually presents with physical symptoms, variant CJD most frequently starts with psychiatric symptoms (mood swings, fatigue, social withdrawal), with physical manifestations appearing some months later.

Clinical features

Acute onset
Disorientation
Speech incoherent, rambling
Memory impairment
Fluctuating conscious level — ↓self awareness
(worse at night) — ↓attention and concentration
↕arousal
Perception
Hallucinations, illusions, distortions (usually visual)
Altered motor activity, occasional aggression;
hypoactive, hyperactive, mixed subtypes
Persecutory delusions common
Autonomic
Sweating, tachycardia, pupillary dilation
Mood
Lability, apathy, perplexity, depression, irritability

Definition

Acute toxic or metabolic,
defect with global,
usually fluctuating,
CNS dysfunction

Incidence

Complicates up to
1/3 of older hospital
admission; more
common in dementia

First-line investigations

Informant history ⎯ alcohol / drugs
Cognitive assesment ⎯ alertness, / memory: recall, orientation / language / visuospatial
Physical examination ⎯ ?infection / ?trauma / focal neurology
Blood
  FBC, ESR, U & E, glucose, LFT, TFT, VDRL, calcium
MSU
Imaging
  CXR, SXR, CT or MRI scan

Aetiology

Predisposing factors	Mechanism
Extremes of age	B lood
Diffuse brain disease	B rain
Cholinergic deficit	B arrier
Dopaminergic exess	B reakdown
Hypercortisolaemia	

Precipitants

Intracranial	Extracranial
Trauma	Infection ⎯ UTI, RTI / septicaemia
Vascular	
TIA	Toxic ⎯ alcohol ⎯ intoxication / withdrawal
Stroke	drugs ⎯ prescribed / illicit
Subdural	
Epilepsy	Endocrine ⎯ ↕thyroid / ↕glycaemia
Infection	Metabolic
Tumour	Uraemia
	↕electrolytes
	Hepatic
	Hypoxia
	Nutritional ↓B1, B12, Folate

Differential diagnosis

Dementia
Depression ⎤ in old age
Mania ⎦
Paraphrenia
Pain, dissociative disorders, response to stress

Delirium	vs.	dementia
Rapid	**Onset**	Gradual
Fluctuating	**Course**	Slowly progressive
Clouded	**Conscious level**	Alert
Abundant incoherent	**Thought content**	Impoverished
Very common esp. visual	**Perceptual abnormalities**	Auditory visual ⎱ 30%

Management

Treat underlying cause
Facilitate orientation
Avoid conflict
Tranquillize sparingly
NB Wernicke's
encephalopathy
(B₁ deficiency) is
medical emergency

Prognosis

Depends on primary cause
Increases length of
hospital stay
Most recover rapidly or die

(handwritten margin notes:)
Drugs:
opiates
Anticonvulsants
L-dopa
Sedatives
post-GA

non convulsive
status (epileptus)
epileptus
post-ictal

The acute confusional state (also known as delirium) is characterized by the rapid onset of a global but fluctuating dysfunction of the central nervous system (CNS), with an underlying toxic, vascular, ictal or metabolic cause. It represents one of the most important problems encountered in liaison psychiatry and is seen by a wide range of specialities, including general and emergency medicine, general and orthopaedic surgery and medicine for the elderly. It may occur in as many as one-third of older patients admitted to hospital either at initial presentation or during hospitalization. It is associated with increased mortality and longer duration of hospitalization.

Clinical features

DSM-IV-TR diagnosis of delirium requires:
1 *Impairment of consciousness and attention.*
2 *Perceptual or cognitive disturbance.* Perceptions – illusions (incorrectly interpreted perceptions) are very common and often frightening; true hallucinations are also common, most frequently visual. Real objects may appear distorted, with size apparently increased or decreased (macro-/micropsia). Cognition – memory and orientation are usually impaired and thinking inefficient; patients complain of being slow and muddled; speech is sometimes incoherent and train of thought is usually difficult to follow. There may be difficulty maintaining attention and distractibility.
3 The disturbance has developed over a *short period of time and fluctuates* (often worse at night – 'sundowning').
4 There is evidence that the delirium may be related to a *physical cause.*
ICD-10 criteria are similar.

Level of arousal may be heightened or decreased. *Motor activity* may be increased but is usually purposeless; aggressive behaviour occurs in about 10% of cases. *Mood* and *affect* may fluctuate rapidly (lability) and be accompanied by irritability or perplexity; apathy and depression are also found. Poorly systematized, transient delusions are common. These may be secondary to abnormal perceptions and are often persecutory, with associated ideas of reference. Sweating, tachycardia and dilated pupils reflect underlying autonomic over-activity. Presentations can be subtle, with patients behaving in an uncharacteristic (e.g. withdrawn, saying little) or bizarre (e.g. demanding hospital discharge in the middle of the night) fashion: underlying disorientation and impaired consciousness may only become apparent on specific inquiry. There may be disturbance of the sleep/wake cycle (e.g. patients may be more alert during the evening and drowsy during the day). Based on the clinical presentation, delirium can be divided into three subtypes: hypoactive (less likely to be recognized), hyperactive and mixed.

Aetiology

Predisposing factors

Delirium is commonest in the very young and the very old. People with diffuse brain disease (dementia or Parkinson's disease) are particularly vulnerable, as are those with deficits in cholinergic neurotransmission or taking drugs with anticholinergic properties (e.g. tricyclic antidepressants, procyclidine). Breakdown of the blood–brain barrier, dopaminergic excess and hypercortisolaemia have all been implicated. Precipitants may be classified as intracranial and extracranial. Among the former are trauma (e.g. boxing injury) and vascular insults, including stroke and haemorrhage, particularly in the subdural space where the presentation may be subacute, and extradurally where sudden collapse may occur after a 'lucid interval'. Epilepsy and intracranial tumour may also present with acute confusion, as may intracranial infection (meningitis, encephalitis or abscess). The so-called great cerebral masqueraders (tuberculosis [TB], neurosyphilis, acquired immunodeficiency syndrome [AIDS]) must always be considered.

A wide range of extracranial pathologies can result in delirium. Infective causes include urinary tract infection (UTI), pneumonia (both of which may be 'silent' in old age with few typical symptoms) and septicaemia. Toxic reactions to drugs frequently cause confusion. Prescribed drugs (including antidepressants, tranquillizers and diuretics) may accumulate in the elderly. Alcohol may confuse both through intoxication (tolerance often decreasing with age) and, most importantly, through withdrawal (delirium tremens [the DTs]). Delirium tremens may occur following abrupt alcohol withdrawal in the context of elective or emergency hospitalization, emphasizing the importance of an accurate alcohol history. Endocrine and metabolic causes of delirium include thyroid hyper- and hypofunction, hyper- and hypoglycaemia (the latter usually more dramatic in onset) and failure of major body systems (heart, lungs, liver, kidneys). Hypoxia is a frequent final common pathway.

Nutritional causes (vitamin B_1, B_{12} or folate deficiency) are uncommon, except when secondary to alcohol abuse. In this context, acute vitamin B_1 deficiency (Wernicke's encephalopathy, characterized by ataxia, ophthalmoplegia, nystagmus and confusion) represents a medical emergency since, if untreated, death or irreversible brain damage (Korsakoff's psychosis, characterized by short-term memory loss and confabulation) occurs.

Differential diagnosis

The diagnosis depends on the demonstration of the cardinal features of delirium (particularly fluctuation in both conscious level and cognitive impairment), the presence of a specific underlying cause and the lack of consistent features of affective or psychotic disorders. Delirium can be particularly difficult to distinguish from dementia (Chapter 32), since people with established dementia are particularly vulnerable to delirium. The distinction from dementia with Lewy bodies, in which cognition typically fluctuates, may be particularly difficult. Delirium should be considered where deterioration has been rapid, the course is fluctuating (rather than slowly progressive), consciousness is clouded rather than alert, and thought content (which in dementia is usually impoverished) is vivid, complex and muddled. Hallucinations occur in both delirium and dementia. In delirium they are very common and predominantly visual; in dementia, on the other hand, they are as frequently auditory and are found in only about one-third of cases.

Other conditions that may resemble delirium are functional psychiatric conditions (mania, depression and late-onset schizophrenia), responses to major stress, particularly severe pain, and dissociative disorders.

Investigations

It is imperative to obtain an informant history, focusing particularly on premorbid level of functioning, onset and course of the confusion and use/abuse of drugs or alcohol. In the mental state assessment, particular attention should be paid to cognitive function (alertness, memory, language, visuospatial ability) and to fluctuation in behaviour. Physical examination is crucial in identifying focal neurological signs and/or evidence of infection or trauma. Appropriate blood investigations for confusion include full blood count (FBC) (to exclude anaemia, macrocytosis, leucocytosis), erythrocyte sedimentation rate (ESR) (infection), urea and electrolytes (U&E) (dehydration, electrolyte imbalance), glucose, thyroid and liver function tests (TFT, LFT), calcium, folate and B_{12} and VDRL (i.e. syphilis serology). Midstream urine (MSU) is mandatory; chest and skull x-rays (CXR, SXR) may be informative. Structural brain imaging (computed tomography [CT] or magnetic resonance imaging [MRI]) and electroencephalography (EEG), where available, can identify many intracranial causes.

Management

A high index of suspicion is essential with patients presenting with an acute onset of altered mental functioning or disturbed behaviour. Specific management should be targeted at detection of the confusional state itself, and at identification and subsequent treatment of underlying pathology. Patients should therefore usually be managed on general hospital (i.e. not psychiatric) wards. General management includes facilitation of orientation. Patients should be nursed in a quiet, well-lit room, avoiding frequent changes in staff (often not possible on general wards). Ensuring they have hearing aids and glasses available, if they need them, and reality orientation (photos of family, a clock or calendar visible) may help. Patients may be very anxious and require consistent explanation and reassurance. Dehydration and electrolyte imbalance are common irrespective of underlying cause, and must be corrected. Aggressive outbursts may be minimized by reassurance and anticipating and avoiding potential conflict. Where undesirable behaviour must be controlled, short-acting benzodiazepines (e.g. lorazepam) are preferable to physical restraint, but should be used sparingly; hypotensive and anticholinergic side-effects may precipitate falls or exacerbate the confusion. Longer-acting benzodiazepines (e.g. diazepam or chlordiazepoxide) are used when the patient is withdrawing from alcohol or drug abuse. Antipsychotics are now avoided where possible due to concerns about increased risk of stroke and mortality when they are prescribed in older people (Chapter 34).

Prognosis

Mortality is high, although dependent on the underlying cause and reduced by rapid diagnosis, identification of any underlying pathology and appropriate general and specific treatment. Where recovery occurs it is usually rapid, with return to premorbid functional level.

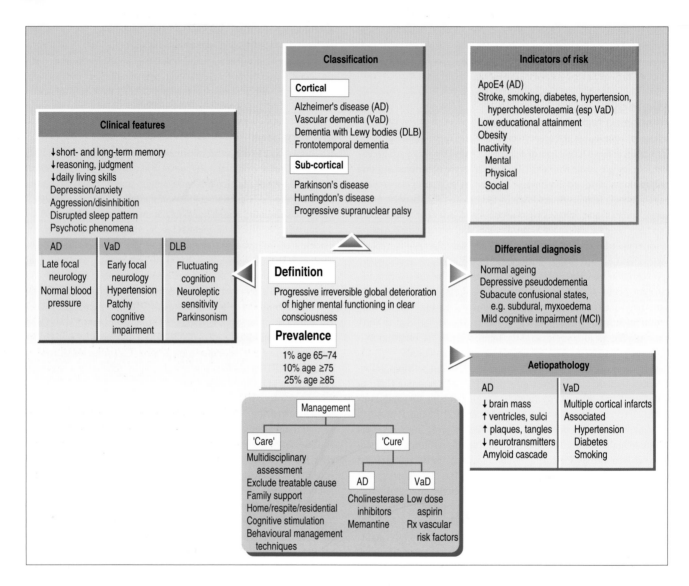

Definition and clinical presentation

Dementia is a syndrome rather than a diagnosis, and refers to a progressive and (usually) irreversible global deterioration of higher cortical functioning in clear consciousness. Symptoms include disruption of memory (short- and long-term), language (nominal aphasia being particularly common), reasoning and judgement. Loss of daily living skills (e.g. washing, dressing, handling money) and abnormal behaviours (e.g. aggression, wandering and sexual disinhibition) can occur. Apathy, depression and anxiety are frequent and there may be disturbances of sleep, including daytime drowsiness, confusion between day and night and nocturnal restlessness. Psychotic phenomena, particularly persecutory delusions (aggravated by forgetfulness) and auditory or, more often, visual hallucinations, occur in one-third of patients. Presentation may occur months or years after the onset of symptoms and is often at family instigation as the person frequently has no insight into the deterioration. The clinical presentation may differ between types of dementia.

Epidemiology

Dementia becomes more common with increasing age. It is rare before the age of 65 but affects 5% of the population aged 65+, 10% aged 75 years and 25% aged 85 years. As the 'old' population in the developing world and the 'very old' population in the developed world increase, the number of people with dementia is projected to rise steeply, as will the burden of providing adequate dementia care. Low educational attainment, obesity, untreated systolic hypertension and mental, social and physical inactivity also increase the risk of late-life dementia.

Classification

The major dementias are degenerative (including Alzheimer's disease and dementia with Lewy bodies [DLB]) or vascular. Dementias are sometimes classified as cortical or subcortical, although the clinical features of both types overlap. Alzheimer's disease, vascular and frontotemporal dementia are examples of cortical dementia; typical symptoms involve memory, language, problem-solving and reasoning. Subcortical dementias occur in Parkinson's disease, Huntington's disease and progressive supra-nuclear palsy; typical symptoms include psychomotor slowing and executive dysfunction associated with disruption to frontal pathways, while focal cognitive symptoms such as aphasia or agnosia are rarely present. Alzheimer's disease is the most frequently diagnosed type of dementia (50–60%), followed by vascular dementia (30%), DLB (<15%) and frontotemporal dementia (<10%).

Alzheimer's disease (AD)

Onset is gradual. At macroscopic level (and on CT and MRI scans), the brain is shrunken, with increased sulcal widening and enlarged ventricles. Microscopically, the key changes are neuronal loss and the presence (particularly in cortex and hippocampus) of *neurofibrillary tangles* and *amyloid plaques*. A protein called *Aβ* is the main constituent of amyloid plaques. The *amyloid cascade hypothesis* states that AD is caused by an imbalance of (too much) brain Aβ production and (too little) Aβ clearance.

Mutations that increase the risk of AD have been identified in three genes: the APP gene and two genes coding for constituents of the secretase enzyme (*presenilin 1* and *presenilin 2*). These account for most cases of familial (early onset) AD, in which inheritance is autosomal dominant. Inheritance of late onset AD is multifactorial and polygenic, the *Apolipoprotein E (ApoE)* gene contributing most to the genetic aetiological component. Three common alleles of ApoE exist (E2, E3, E4); the E4 allele (particularly if homozygous) indicates increased risk and likelihood of earlier onset.

Neurochemically, there are deficits in several neurotransmitters, particularly acetylcholine, noradrenaline, serotonin and somatostatin, with corresponding loss of the cell bodies of neurones secreting these transmitters.

Vascular dementia

This is associated with more patchy cognitive impairment than AD, focal neurological symptoms or signs and a stepwise rather than continuous deterioration. Many people with dementia have a mixed picture of AD and vascular pathology. Pathologically, there are multiple areas of cortical infarction. There is a nine-fold increase in risk of dementia in the year after a stroke. Hypertension, hypercholesterolaemia, diabetes and smoking are risk factors for both vascular dementia and AD.

Dementia with Lewy bodies (DLB)

DLB is characterized by fluctuating cognitive functioning, early visual hallucinations, sensitivity to neuroleptic side-effects and parkinsonism. It is associated with the presence in the basal ganglia and cerebral cortex of Lewy bodies identical to those in the basal ganglia in Parkinson's disease.

About a quarter of people with Parkinson's disease subsequently develop dementia. Where Parkinson's disease pre-dates the dementia by more than a year, the term *Parkinson's disease dementia* (2–4% of all dementias) is used.

Frontotemporal dementia this has a younger mean age of onset and accounts for up to 20% of early onset dementias, but <10% of older onset. It is characterized by early personality changes and relative intellectual sparing. It mainly affects the frontal and anterior temporal lobes.

Alcohol-related dementia accounts for up to 10% of cases.

Normal pressure hydrocephalus this may be idiopathic or due to subarachnoid haemorrhage, head injury or meningitis. It produces a 'patchy' dementia with marked mental slowness, apathy, early onset of wide-based gait and urinary incontinence. Ventriculoatrial shunting may benefit up to 50% of cases.

Dementia may occasionally be associated with repeated head trauma (e.g. boxers), subdural haematoma, or infection (e.g. HIV, syphilis, prion disease) (see Chapters 29–31). Dementias due to metabolic abnormalities (e.g. hyperparathyroidism, hypothyroidism) occur rarely.

Differential diagnosis

Many normal elderly people develop mild, circumscribed deterioration in memory. People without dementia often present with subjective memory problems and can be reassured, though underlying depression should be excluded. Severe depression in old age may present with a pseudodementia, with prominent forgetfulness and poor self-care. Such patients usually have a short history and are often aware of, and distressed by, their poor function. Slowly progressive acute confusional states (e.g. subdural haematoma, myxoedema and vitamin deficiencies) may present with a dementia-like picture. The term mild cognitive impairment (MCI) is used to describe deterioration in cognition insufficient to meet criteria for dementia. People with MCI usually develop dementia.

Management

Controlling vascular risk factors in patients with vascular dementia and prescribing low-dose aspirin reduce the risk of further stroke-related deterioration. Cholinesterase inhibitors (donepezil, rivastigmine, galantamine) can arrest or sometimes temporarily reverse cognitive decline in people with mild to moderate AD and DLB, and may also improve behaviour. Memantine, which modulates glutamate neurotransmission, is licensed for the treatment of moderate to severe AD. No currently available drugs can treat the underlying dementia or prevent it.

Treatment of the neuropsychiatric symptoms is important both for the patient's direct benefit and because they predict caregiver distress and breakdown of care. Patients should have a full assessment to exclude treatable causes and identify specific problems (see Chapter 4 for risk management). The possibility of superimposed and treatable acute confusional states should be considered if a patient deteriorates. Depression often complicates established dementia and may respond to antidepressants.

The focus of management of dementia must be on care delivery, assessing and responding to changing needs, managing risk and maintaining dignity and individuality. Support may include home care input as well as day and intermittent respite. Patients with severe dementia may require residential, nursing or hospital care. Psychological techniques such as cognitive stimulation or teaching behavioural management techniques (see Glossary) to carers may improve cognition and behaviour.

Prognosis

People with dementia die prematurely, even taking into account physical comorbidity. Those who progress to severe dementia usually need full nursing care; death is often from bronchopneumonia. Patients with vascular dementia have a slightly worse prognosis than those with AD.

33 Psychological treatments

Type	Frequency	Number of sessions	Key principles/contents	Main indications
Psychoanalysis	3–5/week	Hundreds	Unconscious defence mechanisms Transference Countertransference Psychological conflicts underlying attachment issues	Personality disorders Psychosexual difficulties Psychosomatic problems
BPP	1–2/week	Variable		

CBT	Weekly	6–12	Negative cognitions
			  Core beliefs
			  Automatic negative thoughts
				Depression
				Anxiety
				Eating disorders
				Schizophrenia
				Some personality disorders

BT	Weekly	6–12	Learning theory Desensitization Operant conditioning Activity schedules	Depression Pain management Recovery after coma or myocardial infarction
DBT	Weekly or more frequent	Variable	Dialectical dilemmas Hierarchy of targets	Borderline personality disorder

IPT	Weekly	12–16	Detailed interpersonal inventory
			Focus on 1 of
			  Role transitions
			  Role disputes
			  Grief and loss
			  Social anxiety
				Depression (non-psychotic)
				Eating disorders

Counselling	Weekly	Variable	Wide range of interventions including
			  Person-centred
			  Non-directive
			  Problem-solving
			  Supportive
				Primary care and medical settings

Psychotherapy seeks to support and sometimes heal through communication between client/patient (CP) and therapist, and the relationship between them. Psychoanalysis and the brief psychological therapies try to help people understand why they feel as they do (how their thinking, relationship style and life-events have affected their current mental state). This understanding can enable them to make changes to the way they interact and perceive the world, and come to terms with past and current stresses. Supportive therapies do not aim to bring about lasting psychological change.

Psychoanalysis

Psychoanalysis stems from the work of Sigmund Freud. Despite considerable modification, the central notion remains that human behaviour is determined predominantly by unconscious forces derived from primitive emotional needs, rather than by reason. Therapy aims to resolve long-standing underlying conflicts and unconscious defence mechanisms (e.g. denial, repression), to promote personal growth and modify the CP's personality by exploring the unconscious, using free association (the CP saying whatever enters his or her mind) and interpretation. The therapist's interpretations make links between events in the CP's history, current life and their relationship with the therapist.

For example, if a CP misses a session immediately following the therapy summer break, the therapist might suggest that the CP felt angry that the therapist had 'abandoned' him or her over the summer and that this evoked memories of an unavailable father in childhood. This might also be linked with a reluctance to commit to current romantic relationships for fear of abandonment.

Sessions are 4–5 times a week for 50 minutes for 2–5 years. Key therapeutic tools are *transference*, where the CP re-experiences strong emotions from early important relationships in their relationship with the therapist; and *countertransference* (the converse) where the therapist experiences strong emotions towards the patient.

Brief psychological therapies
Brief psychodynamic psychotherapy

Related to psychoanalysis. It is an important treatment for those patients with more severe and complex emotional problems, such as personality disorders. It aims to facilitate change by detecting and resolving underlying psychological conflicts or attachment issues which can cause interpersonal problems. Treatment sessions are less frequent than in psychoanalysis (1–2 times a week).

Cognitive–behaviour therapy (CBT)

Depressed patients entertain negatively biased cognitions (thoughts) of themselves, their future and the environment/world (Aaron Beck's cognitive triad). These cognitive distortions (or processing errors) maintain people's negative convictions in the face of contrary evidence. They are thought to arise from underlying beliefs which are the 'rules' or 'silent assumptions' individuals learn from experiences earlier in their lives, often following exposure to traumatic experiences. When exposed to certain stressors at a later date, individuals with abnormal *core (underlying) beliefs* (e.g. 'I am unlovable') are more likely to manifest *automatic negative thoughts* (e.g. 'They are probably not answering the phone because they hate me'). The aim of CBT is initially to help individuals to identify and challenge these automatic thoughts themselves and then to modify any abnormal underlying beliefs. The latter is particularly important if vulnerability to future relapses is to be reduced. For example, a woman who complains that she has no friends might discover that she has a tendency to make automatic presumptions that people find her boring. Perhaps she developed this thinking pattern in childhood in response to a parent who consistently rejected her. Together, the therapist and CP might devise and 'experiment' for her to initiate a conversation with a colleague at work to challenge her negative thoughts.

CBT is also used in the treatment of anxiety, eating disorders, schizophrenia and some personality disorders.

Behaviour therapy (BT)

Based on learning theory. The key tenet is that avoiding feared items, places or actions increases the anxiety associated with them, so creating a vicious cycle. If people challenge their avoidance they will initially become very anxious, but this will eventually decrease (habituation). Techniques include graded exposure to a hierarchy of anxiety-producing situations (systematic desensitization), e.g. to a spider in a glass box, then one on the other side of the room, finally one on the CP's hand. In flooding, the CP is rapidly exposed to an anxiety-producing stimulus. Reciprocal inhibition couples the desensitization with a response incompatible with anxiety (e.g. relaxation, eating). In obsessive–compulsive disorder (OCD), *response prevention* (i.e. stopping compulsive acts, e.g. hand-washing) is important.

Operant conditioning involves encouraging desirable behaviours by positive reinforcement and discouraging undesirable behaviours by withholding reinforcement (negative reinforcement). Negative reinforcement is no longer recommended. Activity schedules to reduce inactivity are often effective in depression, recovery after coma or myocardial infarction, and pain management. Habit reversal training (HRT), used in Tourette's syndrome, aims to increase awareness of tics and develop a competing response to them (e.g. relaxation). Many BT techniques are incorporated into IPT, CBT and DBT (see below).

Interpersonal psychotherapy (IPT)

This is used to treat depression and eating disorders. It focuses on interpersonal aspects of the illness. All close relationships are carefully discussed and any problems conceptualized as difficulties in role transitions (e.g. promotion at work, unemployment, becoming a parent), interpersonal disputes, deficits in the number or quality of relationships, or grief. This formulation is the focus of discussion in subsequent sessions.

Dialectical behaviour therapy (DBT)

This is designed for individuals with borderline personality disorder. The therapy incorporates some components similar to CBT and provides group skills training to equip the individual with alternative coping strategies (rather than deliberate self-harm) when faced with difficulties or emotional instability. The skills taught include mindfulness (bringing one's attention back to the present moment), which is derived from Buddhist meditation.

Mentalization-based treatments

Developed for people with borderline personality disorder, these treatments are based on psychodynamic principles and promote understanding in personal relationships by improving the CPs' ability to deduce the mental states that lie behind their behaviour and that other people.

Group therapy

Emphasizes interrelationships within the group where problems are shared. Groups (of 8–9 members are ideal) meet weekly, and run for months to years. Groups are usually based on psychoanalytic principles; the therapist adopts a non-directive role and uses transference and countertransference processes (see earlier) to make interpretations. CBT is also sometimes delivered in a group format.

Family therapy

May be systemic or behavioural. Systemic theory assumes that problems have arisen with the system of family functioning, not just the individual. It is used predominantly in child and adolescent psychiatry. The expectation is that improved family functioning will result in improvement in the CP.

Milieu therapy

Within an inpatient 'therapeutic community', employs all residents (CPs) and staff to give support to individual CPs, promoting adaptive coping skills and appropriate behaviour by peer pressure. It is most frequently used to treat severe borderline personality disorder that has not responded to other therapies.

Supportive therapies

Counselling and supportive psychotherapy are, in practice, very similar. Duration varies greatly, but is often fairly brief (up to six sessions which help support an individual at times of stress). The therapist works with the CP's symptoms rather than unconscious processes and does not aim at major personality changes. The therapist listens to the CP, seeks to understand the problems and reinforces psychological defence mechanisms. Key components are establishing rapport, facilitating the expression of affect/emotions (e.g. grief, anger), followed by reflection, clarification, reassurance from the therapist, facilitation of the CP's understanding of his or her own feelings and encouragement of problem-solving behaviour. Person-centred counselling, a common form of counselling, is non-directive; the aim is to be with the CP in a meaningful way. Empathy, unconditional positivity and genuineness are the main therapeutic components. As these therapies tend to be unstandardized, their effectiveness is difficult to evaluate, but various forms of supportive therapy have been shown to be effective in primary care and general medical settings.

34 Antipsychotics

Antipsychotics		
Group	Oral	Depot
Phenothiazines	Chlorpromazine Thioridazine Trifluoperazine	Fluphenazine
Butyrophenones	Haloperidol	Haloperidol
Thioxanthenes	Flupentixol Clopenthixol	Flupenthixol Clopenthixol
Diphenylbutyl- piperidines	Pimozide	
Benzamides	Sulpiride Amisulpiride	
Atypical	Clozapine Risperidone Quetiapine Olanzapine Aripiprazole Ziprasidone	

Schizophrenia
Mania
Delusional depression
Tourette's syndrome

Classification

Side-effects

Indications

Side effects	

Antidopaminergic	Movement disorders
	  Parkinsonism
	  Akathisia
	Acute dystonic reactions
	Tardive dyskinesia
	Hyperprolactinaemia

Anticholinergic	Dry mouth Urinary retention Confusion
Antiadrenergic	Postural hypotension Impotence
Antihistaminergic	Sedation
Cardiac	Prolonged QT interval
Toxic	Neuroleptic Malignant Syndrome

The first antipsychotic, chlorpromazine, was introduced in 1951 for anaesthetic (antiemetic) premedication. It was soon tried in schizophrenia and noted to reduce delusions and hallucinations without causing excessive sedation.

Antipsychotics are divided into typical and atypical drugs, the main difference being their side-effect profiles (see below). Atypical antipsychotics are now recommended for first-line treatment of new onset psychosis, but typical antipsychotics are still widely used. The atypical antipsychotics are olanzapine, quetiapine, risperidone, zotepine, clozapine, amisulpiride, ziprasidone and aripiprazole. Typical antipsychotics currently in use are the phenothiazines (chlorpromazine, thioridazine, fluphenazine and trifluoperazine), the butyrophenones (haloperidol), the thioxanthenes (flupentixol, zuclopenthixol), the diphenylbutylpiperidines (pimozide) and the substituted benzamides (sulpiride). Only clozapine has demonstrated superior efficacy, but because of its potentially dangerous side-effects (see later) is prescribed only after two different antipsychotics have failed to control symptoms.

Mechanism of action

Typical antipsychotics are dopamine-receptor blockers but also block cholinergic, adrenergic and histaminergic receptors. Atypical antipsychotics also block dopamine receptors, usually with a lower affinity; in addition they are 5HT$_2$ antagonists. They have relatively little activity on other receptors. Older drugs (phenothiazines) are relatively non-selective, whereas sulpiride and amisulpiride are highly selective blockers of D2 dopamine receptors.

Mode of administration

This is usually by mouth, with extensive first-pass metabolism in the liver. Many can also be given by short-acting intramuscular (IM) or (very rarely) intravenous injection. Some (such as flupentixol [Depixol], fluphenazine [Modecate] and risperidone [Risperdal]) can be given by depot injection every 1–4 weeks. This bypasses first-pass metabolism; it may improve adherence (and therefore prevent relapse) or at least allow closer monitoring.

Indications

Treatment and relapse prevention in schizophrenia and other psychoses (e.g. mania, psychotic depression in combination with antidepressants); they are most effective in alleviating positive symptoms such as delusions, hallucinations and thought disorder. Clozapine and amisulpiride may be more effective against negative symptoms (see Chapter 6) than other neuroleptics. Antipsychotics are also used to treat Tourette's syndrome and some atypical antipsychotics (risperidone, olanzapine and quetiapine) are licensed for treatment of acute mania. Atypical antipsychotics are no longer recommended for treatment of violent or agitated behaviour in older people with dementia because of the increased risk of stroke and impairment of glycaemic control.

Side-effects

Patients report that movement disorders, sedation, weight gain and sexual dysfunction are the most troublesome side-effects of antipsychotics. Weight gain (especially with clozapine and olanzapine) and impaired glucose tolerance and diabetes mellitus are particularly associated with atypical antipsychotics. Clozapine may cause potentially fatal agranulocytosis and seizures, and requires regular haematological monitoring.

Due to their more potent dopaminergic effects, typical antipsychotics are more likely than atypical antipsychotics to cause extrapyramidal movement disorders (due to reduced dopamine availability in the nigrostriatal pathways) and raised prolactin, leading to endocrine effects (secondary to tubero-infundibular dopamine blockade). Both typical and atypical antipsychotics can cause anti-cholinergic, anti-adrenergic, anti-histaminergic and cardiac side-effects.

Movement disorders include acute dystonic reactions (torticollis, oculogyric crisis, increased muscle tone), parkinsonism symptoms or akathisia (psychomotor restlessness). Acute dystonia and parkinsonism reflect drug-induced dopamine/acetylcholine imbalance and respond to anticholinergic drugs such as procyclidine. Akathisia is less responsive to anticholinergics; beta-blockers or benzodiazepines may be helpful. Akathisia may lead to suicide. Long-term antipsychotics may cause tardive dyskinesia (TD), thought to be due to dopamine-receptor supersensitivity and characterized by abnormal buccolingual masticatory movements and, in severe cases, choreiform trunk and limb movements, especially in older people. Tetrabenazine may reduce the movements of TD as may reduction or cessation of antipsychotics, although it is irreversible in 50% of cases. Procyclidine does not help TD and may make it worse. *Endocrine effects* include hyperprolactinaemia and consequent amenorrhoea, galactorrhoea and sexual dysfunction.

Anticholinergic effects include dry mouth, confusion and urinary retention. *Antiadrenergic effects* include postural hypotension and impotence. *Histaminegric blockade* causes sedation. Toxic effects include the neuroleptic malignant syndrome (hyperpyrexia, autonomic instability, confusion and increased muscle tone, raised serum creatine (CPK) phosphokinase); and (with phenothiazines) blood dyscrasias, retinal pigmentation, photosensitivity and cholestatic jaundice. Antipsychotics may also be an associated with prolonged ECG QT interval and arrhythmia.

Chlorpromazine - EPS, antidopamine + ↑prolactin. very sedative

TCAs - Amitriptyline - anticholinergic

Haloperidol - Neuroleptic malignant syndrome - Rx cooling + dantrolene (most commonly)

Fluphenazine - less sedative, less antichol, ↑↑EPS

Clozapine - agranulocytosis ∴ only use if not responded to other drugs in schizophrenia

Amisulpiride + Quetiapine - less daytime sedation

Quetiapine, olanzapine, aripirazole - small ↑prolactin

Amisulpiride + risperidone - ↓weight gain than others, also ↓ glucose int'l / dyslipidaemia

Typical → less effective on -ve symptoms

D2 receptor block → (mesolimbic system) cortex, limbic system → sedation } Anti-psychotic, impaired performance
↓ nigrostriatal - basal (striatum) ganglia - movement disorders - acute dystonia, akathisia, parkinsonism, TD
↓ Tubero-infundibular - pituitary - ↑prolactin - gynaecomastia, galactorrhoea, menstrual irregularities, impotence, weight gain

Indications
Moderate or severe depressive episode or relapse prevention OCD, PTSD, anxiety and panic disorders, bulimia nervosa

▽

Antidepressant	Side effects	
SSRIs Fluoxetine Citalopram Paroxetine Sertraline Fluvoxamine **SNRIs** Venlafaxine Duloxetine	Headache Anorexia Nausea Indigestion Anxiety Sexual dysfunction ⚠ ↑ suicide ideation; not recommended < 18 years (except fluoxetine) ⚠ withdrawal syndrome	**SSRIs only:** ⚠ Gastrointestinal bleeding Hyponatraemia in older people *SIADH* **Venlafaxine:** Hypertension / hypotension Cardiotoxic in overdose
NaSSA Mirtazapine	Dry mouth, drowsiness and weight gain	
TCIs Amitriptyline Dothiepin Imipramine Lofepramine	Anticholinergic Antiadrenergic ⚠ cardiac arrhythmias ⚠ seizures	
MAOI Phenelzine Tranylcypromine	Anticholinergic Antiadrenergic Tyramine reaction — *Hypertensive crisis*	

MAO-A reversible inhibitor - moclobamide
Noradrenaline selective reuptake inhibitor - Reboxetine

Selective serotonin reuptake inhibitors (SSRIs) (citalopram, fluvoxamine, fluoxetine, sertraline and paroxetine) were introduced in the 1980s and are now the most commonly prescribed class of antidepressants in the developed world. Drugs introduced more recently are the reversible inhibitor of MAO-A, moclobemide; venlafaxine and duloxetine (selective serotonin and noradrenaline reuptake inhibitors [SNRIs]); mirtazapine, which has a noradrenergic and selective serotonergic action; and the noradrenaline selective reuptake inhibitor reboxetine. Other antidepressants available include trazodone, maprotiline, mianserin and nefazodone. The herbal preparation hypericum (St John's wort), whose active ingredient is thought to be hypericin, is widely used and may be effective in mild to moderate depression. Its action is similar to that of monoamine oxidase inhibitors (MAOIs); it may interact adversely with many other drugs.

Antidepressants available prior to 1980 were divided into the tricyclics (such as imipramine, amitriptyline, dothiepin and lofepramine) and the MAOIs (e.g. phenelzine and tranylcypromine). Tricyclic antidepressants are still in regular use, while MAOIs are only occasionally prescribed.

Mechanism of action

The common mechanism of action of antidepressants involves modulation of pre- and/or postsynaptic receptors or electrophysiological responses to increase availability of serotonin and noradrenaline in the synaptic cleft. This may then produce an antidepressant effect, probably through up-regulation of brain-derived neurotrophic factors (BDNFs), which are down-regulated by increased levels of cortisol produced at times of stress. Tricyclics and SNRIs block reuptake of both noradrenaline and serotonin into the presynaptic neurone; SSRIs have a similar action on serotonin alone. MAOIs inhibit the breakdown of serotonin (and to a lesser extent noradrenaline) at the synapse by inhibition of MAO-A. Mianserin and mirtazapine block presynaptic α_2-receptors.

Mode of administration

This is by mouth. Most antidepressants can be given once daily and are extensively and variably metabolized by first pass in the liver. The antidepressant response seldom occurs in less than two weeks and may not be fully apparent for six weeks, though early partial response is predictive of remission. Patients not warned of the delayed therapeutic action are likely to be less treatment-adherent.

Indications

The main indication for antidepressants is a moderate or severe depressive episode. Patients with biological features of depression are most likely to respond. Studies suggest a response rate of 60–70% (compared to 30% with placebo). Antidepressants are also useful in phobic anxiety, panic disorder, bulimia nervosa, post-traumatic stress disorder (PTSD), general anxiety disorder (GAD), obsessive–compulsive disorder (OCD), in which higher doses may be needed, and in preventing depressive relapse.

Side-effects

SSRIs and SNRIs may cause headache, anorexia, nausea, indigestion, anxiety (although in many they are anxiolytic) or sexual dysfunction. SSRIs have been associated with an increased risk of gastrointestinal bleeding, especially in older people, so should be avoided if possible in patients aged over 80 years, those with prior upper GI bleeding and in those taking aspirin or a non-steroidal anti-inflammatory

drug. SSRIs may occasionally cause hyponatraemia in older people. [*SIADH*] There is increasing recent evidence that SSRIs and SNRIs may increase agitation during the first 1–2 weeks of use, and may also be associated with dysphoria and a range of unpleasant withdrawal phenomena if stopped abruptly. Gradual tapering over 2–4 weeks is recommended. There have been some reports that SSRIs and venlafaxine may be associated with increased suicidal ideation and aggression, and due to these concerns all except fluoxetine are contraindicated in children under 18. Venlafaxine may cause hypertension (or hypotension); while SSRIs are very safe in overdose, venlafaxine is associated with greater risks from cardiotoxicity. The commonest side-effects of mirtazapine are dry mouth, drowsiness and weight gain.

Tricyclic side-effects include anticholinergic and antiadrenergic effects similar to those of the antipsychotics. In overdose they may trigger potentially fatal cardiac arrhythmias and seizures. Lofepramine is relatively safe in overdose and free of anticholinergic effects. MAOIs (not moclobemide) can cause an occasionally fatal syndrome of hypertension and throbbing headache if foods containing large quantities of tyramine (e.g. cheese, red wine) are eaten.

36 Other psychotropic drugs

Antimanic agents	Sedatives
Uses	
Treating acute mania (Lithium only)	Insomnia
Prophylaxis in bipolar disorder	Anxiety
Refractory depression	Alcohol withdrawal
	Control of violence
Side effects	
Lithium: nausea, tremor, weight gain, polydipsia	Drowsiness
Carbemazapine: nausea, drowiness, dizziness, blood dyscrasias	Ataxia
Valproic acid: nausea, gastric irritation, diarrhoea, weight gain	
Warnings	
Teratogenic	Dependency
Lithium has narrow therapeutic window; blood monitoring essential	Paradoxical aggression
Carbamazepine may affect metabolism of other drugs	

Antimanic drugs

Lithium is the archetypal mood stabilizer. It is used for prophylaxis in recurrent affective disorder (unipolar and bipolar), acute treatment of mania and augmentation of antidepressants in resistant depression. There is evidence that lithium reduces the risk of suicide. It may also be used in schizoaffective illness and in the control of aggression. For prophylaxis in bipolar affective disorder, carbamazepine (which may be particularly useful in rapid cycling bipolar illness), valproic acid and lamotrigine are also used.

Mode of administration

Lithium is taken by mouth and excreted by the kidneys. It has a narrow therapeutic range (0.4–1.0 mmol/L). Prior to commencing lithium therapy, thyroid and renal function should be evaluated. Serum lithium levels should be monitored regularly (initially weekly, thereafter every 12 weeks), and blood taken 8–12 hours after last dose. In patients on lithium, renal and thyroid function tests, and in those on carbamazepine full blood count (FBC), should be monitored every six months. Patients on carbamazepine should be warned that an unexplained sore throat may herald agranulocytosis.

Mechanism of action

Lithium interacts with all biological systems where sodium, potassium, calcium or magnesium are involved. At therapeutic blood levels it probably has effects on neurotransmission, including 5HT, noradrenaline, dopamine and acetylcholine. Its interference with cyclic adenosine monophosphate (cAMP)-linked receptors explains its action on the thyroid and kidney.

Side-effects and toxic effects

Side-effects of lithium include nausea, fine tremor, weight gain, oedema, polydipsia, polyuria, exacerbation of psoriasis and acne, and hypothyroidism. Toxicity is indicated by vomiting, diarrhoea, coarse tremor, slurred speech, ataxia, drowsiness, confusion, convulsions and coma. Treatment of toxicity/overdose involves cessation of lithium, forced diuresis (intravenous mannitol), haemodialysis or peritoneal dialysis. Carbamazepine may cause blood dyscrasias and rashes and may alter blood levels of other drugs metabolized by the same cytochrome P450 pathways. Common side-effects of valproic acid are nausea, gastric irritation, diarrhoea and weight gain. Diabetes insipidus

Contraindications

Lithium should be avoided in renal, cardiac, thyroid and Addison's disease and in pregnancy and breastfeeding. Dehydration and diuretics can lead to lithium toxicity. Adverse interactions can also occur between lithium and non-steroidal anti-inflammatory drugs, calcium channel blockers and some antibiotics. Carbamazepine is also teratogenic and may interfere with the action of oral contraceptives, necessitating other contraceptive precautions.

Sedatives

The most commonly used are the *benzodiazepines* (BDZs), zopiclone and related compounds. As the BDZs are anxiolytic, sleep-inducing, anticonvulsant and muscle-relaxant, their indications include insomnia, generalized (but not phobic) anxiety, alcohol withdrawal states and the control of violent behaviour. Underlying conditions (e.g. depression) should always be excluded and behavioural alternative treatments considered. BDZs are also used as second-line drugs in refractory epilepsy.

Zopiclone and zolpidem are commonly used hypnotics; sedative antihistamines such as promethazine are available over the counter in Britain. Buspirone has anxiolytic effects.

Mode of administration

Usually oral, but intramuscular, intravenous or rectal administration may be required in status epilepticus and in violent patients.

Pharmacokinetics

Most have active metabolites, some with a half-life of several days. The long-acting BDZs include diazepam, chlordiazepoxide and nitrazepam; lorazepam, oxazepam and temazepam are shorter-acting BDZs.

Mechanism of action

With the exception of antihistamines, they potentiate the inhibitory effects of γ-aminobutyric acid (GABA).

Toxic effects and side-effects

Drowsiness, sedation, ataxia, respiratory depression and disinhibition, which may lead (paradoxically) to aggression. Tolerance to BDZs frequently occurs, and there is a prolonged withdrawal syndrome, with marked anxiety, shakiness, abdominal cramps, perceptual disturbances, persecutory delusions and fits. They should therefore usually be prescribed for no more than a couple of weeks. Weaning patients off BDZs to which they have (iatrogenically) become dependent may take months or even years. BDZs potentiate alcohol and other sedatives; the combination is dangerous in overdose. Zopiclone and related compounds may also cause dependency; long-term use should therefore be avoided.

Electroconvulsive therapy (ECT) and other treatments

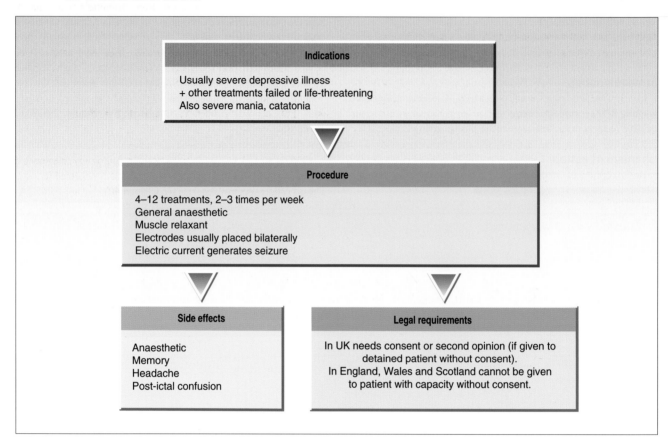

Indications

Usually severe depressive illness
+ other treatments failed or life-threatening
Also severe mania, catatonia

Procedure

4–12 treatments, 2–3 times per week
General anaesthetic
Muscle relaxant
Electrodes usually placed bilaterally
Electric current generates seizure

Side effects

Anaesthetic
Memory
Headache
Post-ictal confusion

Legal requirements

In UK needs consent or second opinion (if given to detained patient without consent).
In England, Wales and Scotland cannot be given to patient with capacity without consent.

ECT

Mechanism of action

ECT involves the induction of a modified epileptic seizure. A series of such treatments induces complex effects, including neurotransmitter release, a transient increase in blood–brain barrier permeability, secretion of hypothalamic and pituitary hormones, and modulation of neurotransmitter receptors similar to those induced by antidepressant drugs.

Mode of administration

ECT is given 2–3 times a week, usually up to a total of 4–12 treatments. Before each treatment the patient is fasted for at least four hours and is then given a short-acting anaesthetic, a muscle-relaxant drug and a few seconds' pre-oxygenation prior to the application of an electric current sufficient to trigger an epileptic seizure. This is given through electrodes placed bitemporally or with both on the non-dominant hemisphere.

Legal aspects

In England and Wales, ECT can only be given if either the patient has given informed consent or is detained under the Mental Health Act 1983 (MHA) and an independent consultant appointed by the Mental Health Act Commission agrees that ECT must be given. In the latter situation, ECT can be initiated prior to the independent consultant's assessment under the provisions of section 62 of the Act. Under the 2007 MHA, ECT may only be given without consent if the patient is judged to lack capacity to consent. Legal aspects of ECT in Scotland and Ireland are covered in Chapter 41.

Indications

The UK National Institute for Clinical Excellence (NICE) recommends that ECT should only be used for the treatment of severe depressive illness (the main indication), a prolonged or severe episode of mania, or catatonia. They state that ECT should be used to induce rapid and short-term improvement of severe symptoms after all other treatment options have failed, or when the situation is thought to be life-threatening (due to high risk of suicide or not eating and drinking). Patients with depressive delusions and/or psychomotor retardation are likeliest to respond. Response rates may be as high as 90%. Speed of response may be faster than that of antidepressants.

Contraindications

There are no absolute contraindications to ECT. Raised intracranial pressure, recent stroke or myocardial infarction and crescendo angina are important relative contraindications.

Side-effects

Side-effects include anaesthetic complications, dysrhythmias due to vagal stimulation, post-ictal headache and confusion and retro-

and anterograde amnesia with difficulties in registration and recall that may persist for several weeks. Memory problems are reduced by unilateral electrode placement which may, however, be slightly less effective.

Eye movement desensitization and reprocessing (EMDR)

EMDR is a psychotherapy treatment which aims to help patients access and process traumatic memories with the goal of emotionally resolving them. During EMDR the client attends to emotionally disturbing material while simultaneously focusing on an external stimulus. This stimulus usually involves the therapist directing the patient's lateral eye movements by asking them to look first one way then the other. There is evidence that EMDR is an effective treatment for post-traumatic stress disorder.

New methods of brain stimulation

Transcranial magnetic stimulation (TMS; the prefrontal cortex is stimulated by the application of a strong magnetic field) has shown promise in the treatment of depression, OCD and Tourette's syndrome (TS). Vagal nerve stimulation (VNS) is used in epilepsy and has antidepressant effects. In deep brain stimulation (DBS) a thin electrode is inserted directly into the brain and currents applied. It has been used in Parkinson's disease, OCD and TS. None of these techniques is yet established in clinical practice outside the USA.

Neurosurgery for mental disorder

This is now extremely rare (<10 operations a year in UK). Indications are severe depression and obsessive compulsive disorder. Success rates of 40–60% are reported. Bilateral anterior capsulotomy or anterior cingulotomy are the only two procedures currently performed in the UK. The procedure requires consent (see Chapter 40).

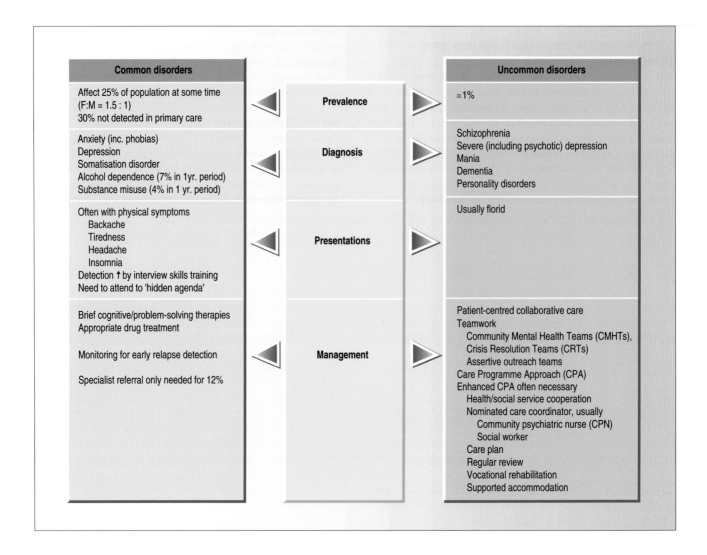

Common disorders		Uncommon disorders
Affect 25% of population at some time (F:M = 1.5 : 1) 30% not detected in primary care	Prevalence	≃1%
Anxiety (inc. phobias) Depression Somatisation disorder Alcohol dependence (7% in 1yr. period) Substance misuse (4% in 1 yr. period)	Diagnosis	Schizophrenia Severe (including psychotic) depression Mania Dementia Personality disorders
Often with physical symptoms Backache Tiredness Headache Insomnia Detection ↑ by interview skills training Need to attend to 'hidden agenda'	Presentations	Usually florid
Brief cognitive/problem-solving therapies Appropriate drug treatment Monitoring for early relapse detection Specialist referral only needed for 12%	Management	Patient-centred collaborative care Teamwork Community Mental Health Teams (CMHTs), Crisis Resolution Teams (CRTs) Assertive outreach teams Care Programme Approach (CPA) Enhanced CPA often necessary Health/social service cooperation Nominated care coordinator, usually Community psychiatric nurse (CPN) Social worker Care plan Regular review Vocational rehabilitation Supported accommodation

Most patients with mental illness are managed in primary care (if their illness is detected at all). Only those with severe and enduring mental illness are treated by psychiatric services, the great majority remaining in the community rather than being admitted to hospital.

Psychiatry in primary care

Community surveys in the UK and USA suggest that about 25% of the population aged 18–65 years experience significant psychiatric morbidity at one time, most frequently anxiety or depression. Women outnumber men by a factor of about 1.5. Approximately 15% of people in Britain report ever considering suicide. Dependence on alcohol or other drugs (7% and 4% respectively within a one-year period) and personality disorder (5%) are relatively less common in the general population, although both are common in people presenting to psychiatric services. Psychoses are also relatively rare (<1%). In older people, the total prevalence of psychiatric illness is particularly high because of the age-associated rise in the prevalence of dementia (Chapter 32).

In the UK, most people are registered with a general practitioner (GP), and psychiatric morbidity doubles the likelihood of GP consulta-

tion. One in four GP consultations relates to mental health. About 30% of significant psychiatric illness is not detected by primary care. Illness is less likely to be detected (and therefore successfully treated) in patients who do not accept that their illness is psychiatric or treatable, or do not perceive their GP as sympathetic or understanding. Cultural differences in the way that people express mental illness can also affect detection rates in primary care. GP training, attitudes and time available for consultation may also contribute. Detection rates may be increased by improved communication skills, including appropriate use of eye contact, sensitivity to non-verbal cues and avoiding exclusive concentration on the presenting complaint at the expense of any 'hidden agenda'. The most common psychiatric illnesses among people attending primary care are depression, anxiety and somatization disorder (Chapter 27).

Only about one-eighth of cases detected will be referred to psychiatrists. The decision to refer may reflect the GP's confidence in managing psychiatric illness, the patient's wishes, the accessibility of the psychiatric service, and the severity and duration of the illness. The challenge of primary care psychiatry is to ensure recognition and optimal care for

82 *Psychiatry at a Glance*, 4e. By C. Katona, C. Cooper and M. Robertson. Published 2008 Blackwell Publishing. ISBN: 978-1-4501-8117-4

the 'submerged iceberg' of psychiatric morbidity. Brief cognitive or problem-solving therapies are effective treatments for depression and anxiety, but are more time-consuming than medication, and the demand for them currently exceeds their availability. It is therefore often quicker and easier to prescribe medication than deliver psychological therapies, even when these would be more appropriate. *Primary mental health care workers* are now employed in some areas to deliver these therapies within primary care. Most *community mental health teams* (CMHTs) have formal arrangements for liaison with local GP surgeries (e.g. regular meetings to discuss joint care). Many Foundation and GP training rotations now include a six-month post in psychiatry.

Community care of severe psychiatric illness

Between 1980 and 1995, large psychiatric hospitals (asylums) closed and the majority of psychiatric care shifted to the community, supported by fewer, smaller inpatient units. This radical change was enabled by the effectiveness of psychotropic drugs, as well as an ideological commitment to the closure of asylums and reductions in bed numbers as a cost-cutting exercise. Since 2000, the number of inpatient beds has declined further as *crisis resolution teams* (CRTs, sometimes called home treatment teams) have been set up to manage severely unwell people at home. With the closure of beds and introduction of home treatment, the psychiatric inpatient population has changed markedly. Only those with the severest illness or highest risk are found on inpatient wards and a large proportion are detained under the Mental Health Act.

Most secondary psychiatric care is now delivered by CMHTs, comprised of psychiatrists, community psychiatric nurses (CPNs), social workers, occupational therapists (OTs) and psychologists. General adult CMHTs care for people aged 18–65, older people's CMHTs for people aged 65+, and child and adolescent services for people aged under 18.

Dedicated teams work with people who are acutely unwell or reluctant to engage with services. CRTs provide intensive support for people in mental health crises in their own home. The team operates 24 hours a day, and sees people very frequently, sometimes twice a day, with the aim of preventing admissions and supporting early discharge.

Assertive outreach teams (AOTs) provide intensive treatment and support in the community for people who are chronically unwell and who have a history of disengagement from mainstream services. *Early intervention in psychosis services* (EIS) have been set up in many areas to work with patients, usually between the ages of 18 and 35, who are newly diagnosed with psychosis. They provide intensive treatment for the first 2–3 years of illness, with the aim of promoting recovery in the early stages of psychotic illness, when evidence suggests treatment might be more effective, with a focus on promoting return to employment and education.

Psychiatric care is managed through the *care programme approach* (CPA) in England, Wales and Scotland (introduced by the Community Care Act 1991). In Northern Ireland, care plans are reviewed on a regular basis in a similar system. CPA meetings take place at least six-monthly to devise a care plan, documenting all those involved in the patient's care, their treatment plan, early relapse indicators and a crisis plan should their mental health deteriorate. The patient, usually their family and all relevant professionals and services (primarily the health and social services but also housing, GP) are invited. Each patient has a nominated *care coordinator* (who may be any member of the CMHT), who arranges the CPA and is responsible for the care plan, seeing patients regularly (usually monthly). The care coordinator also monitors the patient's mental state and medication adherence, detecting any relapses at an early stage, providing emotional and practical support and promoting the patient's mental well-being (e.g. by avoiding stress, excessive alcohol and drug use).

There are two CPA levels: *standard CPA*, for people requiring input from one health professional and who do not pose a risk to themselves or others; and *enhanced CPA* for those with psychotic or more severe affective disorders, indicating they are likely to require the services of more than one professional (e.g. GP and social worker).

Services aim to provide patient-centred collaborative care, involving patients and their families in treatment decisions, reflecting a shift from previous 'paternalistic' services. Many patients find self-help groups beneficial. Service users (patients) are increasingly involved in the management of services, training professionals and advising current patients through 'patient advocacy' services.

Patients unable to live independently may be cared for by family or friends (who may themselves need support from services to provide this care). Supported accommodation projects such as group homes or hostels are usually run by Social Services or voluntary organizations; the amount of professional support can vary from 24-hour nursing staff to mental health workers visiting two or three times a week. Most aim to provide rehabilitation so that people can return to independent living or less supported settings. The assessment of individuals' ability to care for themselves (personal hygiene, shopping, budgeting, cooking, cleaning) and the nature of their illness are important in deciding what level of support they will need to live successfully in the community and avoid relapse and return to hospital.

Employment provides income, purpose, structure and social networks. Unemployment is associated with poverty, stress, low self-esteem and depression. Barriers to people with mental illness staying in employment or returning to work include lack of motivation, anxiety, concerns about losing state benefits and discrimination, although the Disability Discrimination Act 1995 prohibits employers from treating people with chronic (including mental) illness differently.

Most services now focus on supporting people with mental health problems to obtain employment, attend college courses or train for work. *Day centres* (run by health and social care or voluntary services) provide structured daytime activity for those whose disabilities prevent them from achieving mainstream employment. Their focus is on developing service users' occupational skills so that they can gain access to higher education and voluntary or mainstream employment and providing social support and access to leisure pursuits. *Support, time and recovery* (STaR) workers employed by these and other services facilitate service users to access a range of daytime activities.

Testamentary capacity

Ability to make a will requires
Understanding of
    What a will is
    What its consequences are
    Nature/extent of own property
    Identity/claims of potential beneficiaries
Judgement not distorted by mental illness

Fitness to plead

Requires
    Understanding of
        Nature of charges
        Meaning of guilty/not guilty plea
    Capacity to
        Instruct counsel
        Challenge jurors
        Follow court proceedings/evidence

Mens rea (guilty mind)

Necessary for conviction of most offences
Insufficient if
    Aged < 10 (*doli incapax*)
    Not guilty by reason of insanity
    Diminished responsibility
    Incapacity to form an intent (automatism)

Legal competence

Lack of capacity

Situation-specific inability to understand, use and retain relevant information to come to a decision and communicate decision

Mental Capacity Act 2005 (England and Wales)

If person lacks capacity to make decision about health, welfare, property:
- Must act in best interests
- Duty to consult relatives
- Appoint independent mental capacity advocate (IMCA) for serious decisions if no family/close friend to consult

A person with capacity can make provisions for losing capacity:
- Appoint lasting power of attorney
- Advance decision

Crime and mental disorder

Diagnosis	Associated criminal activity
Depression	Shoplifting Murder followed by suicide
Schizophrenia	Shoplifting Damage to property Violence rare
Alcohol/drug abuse	Theft Driving offences Violence
Learning disability	Sexual offences Arson
Antisocial personality disorder	Rape Shoplifting Homicide
Mania	Fraud Defaulted debt
Dementia	Shoplifting Sexual offences

Forensic psychiatry concerns the legal aspects of mental disorders. The forensic psychiatrist is primarily concerned with the assessment, treatment and rehabilitation of mentally disordered offenders.

Crime and mental disorder

Psychiatric illnesses, particularly psychoses and drug- or alcohol-related disorders, are overrepresented in prisoners. This partly reflects a group of urban, homeless, psychiatrically ill, multiple reoffenders (see Chapter 24). The overall rate of offending by people with a mental illness appears similar to that in the general population, although mental disorder may increase the likelihood of arrest. Specific associations have, however, been demonstrated between offences and psychiatric diagnoses.

Patients with *schizophrenia* often commit minor offences such as shoplifting or damage to property. Violence is rare and usually domestic, and occurs in response to poor tolerance of family stress. The specific and much publicized link with homicide is usually in the context of florid psychosis secondary to poor treatment compliance.

Depression may be heralded by a minor 'out-of-character' offence (e.g. shoplifting). Depression-related homicide is rare, usually domestic (typically infanticide), often in response to delusions (e.g. believing that the victim is fatally ill and suffering) and frequently followed by suicide. Offences linked to *mania* (fraud, defaulted debt) usually reflect financial irresponsibility.

Alcohol and substance misuse are associated with theft, robbery, assault and homicide. Acute alcohol intoxication weakens inhibitions against offending ('Dutch courage') and is strongly linked with driving offences. Theft and robbery may also be motivated by a lack of funds to buy illicit drugs. Alcohol is often implicated in *morbid* or *pathological jealousy* (see Chapter 18) which may culminate in spousal homicide.

Dementia is occasionally associated with shoplifting (forgetting to pay) and sexual offences (usually reflecting frontal disinhibition). Similarly, subjects with *learning disability* (see Chapter 24) may commit sexual offences or arson. Violent acts may be committed by younger, brain-damaged subjects unable to handle stress or frustration.

The link between crime and personality disorder is complex: the association between crime and *antisocial personality disorder* is somewhat circular, since offending may be integral to the diagnosis. Individuals with long-standing paranoid characteristics, people who cannot control their anger and those with severe impulsive and histrionic traits are all more likely than others to offend.

Predictors of violence in offenders

Most mentally ill people are never dangerous, and most violent crimes are committed by people without mental illness. Assessment of risk is important when assessing for compulsory detention, transferring patients between different levels of security and planning aftercare. Crimes against property and violence against the person need to be distinguished. While a history of violence is a strong predictor of future risk (see Chapter 4), a first episode of violence can occur in the context of severe stress or a psychotic disorder. An offender who has a past history of violence must be monitored carefully, with special reference to recurrence of previous precursors. Risk may have to be managed by compulsory detention, sometimes long-term. Resource issues should not be allowed to cloud judgements about the management of violence.

Legal competence

Most mentally ill people retain responsibility for their actions and the capacity to manage their affairs. There are, however, circumstances where careful assessment of capacity is crucial.

Fitness to plead is for a jury to decide and refers to a defendant's competence to mount a defence against charges. A person is deemed fit to plead if they have the mental capacity to understand the charge, distinguish between guilty and not guilty pleas, instruct lawyers, follow court evidence and challenge jurors. A trial of the facts may nonetheless take place, with acquittal if the facts are not established and flexibility of sentence if proven.

For guilt (of most crimes) to be established, it is necessary to demonstrate that the defendant was 'criminally responsible', possessing the *mens rea* (MR) (guilty mind) to commit the offence. MR may be absent by virtue of age, psychiatric illness or automatism and lack of criminal intent (e.g. accidents). Children under 10 years of age cannot be held criminally responsible, and for those aged 10–14 years the prosecution must prove MR. Mental disorder is rarely invoked to deny MR; it must be established that the defendant was mentally ill at the time of the offence, resulting in a 'defect of reason or disease of the mind', and that in consequence the verdict is 'not guilty by reason of insanity'. This theoretically allows some flexibility of sentence, although it usually results in hospital detention. 'Automatism' refers to dissociation between mind and action (e.g. epilepsy, sleepwalking, concussion).

In murder, conviction may be modified to manslaughter on grounds of *diminished responsibility* on the basis of specific 'abnormality of mind' substantially impairing mental responsibility. This is defined as 'arising from a condition of arrested or retarded development of mind or any inherent causes or induced by disease or injury'.

Testamentary capacity (TC; competence to make a will) must be present for a will to be valid. It requires a person to understand the act of making a will; to appreciate the extent of his or her property and assets; and to be aware of who might have a reasonable claim on his or her estate. If the person is mentally ill, TC implies that his/her judgement should not be clouded regarding the will itself. Delusions or hallucinations only impair TC where they are directly relevant to the will (e.g. delusions of poverty).

The Mental Capacity Act (England and Wales)

Lack of capacity may be due to any cause (temporary or permanent) that impairs reasoning ability (e.g. dementia, intellectual disability, acute confusional state). A person lacks capacity to make a decision if he or she is unable to understand information relevant to the decision, retain, use and weigh that information to come to a decision, and communicate that decision (by talking, sign language or other means). If a lack of capacity is likely to be temporary, it may be possible to delay the decision until the person regains capacity, otherwise professionals must make decisions in their best interests. They have a duty to consult carers and family. If the person has no one to speak for them, an Independent Mental Capacity Advocate (IMCA) is appointed to represent their wishes.

The Mental Capacity Act allows a person with capacity to appoint an attorney to make these decisions on their behalf if they should lose capacity in the future (*Lasting Power of Attorney*). Attorneys can be directed by the person appointing them to make decisions on their behalf covering property and financial affairs, and personal welfare (which includes health care). The Act also permits anyone with capacity to make an *advance decision* about treatment that they do not want to receive in the future if they lose capacity to make treatment decisions. Advance decisions permit a person to refuse treatment but not to demand treatment.

The Adults with Incapacity (Scotland) Act 2000

This sets out similar legislation for appointing a Power of Attorney to look after personal property and financial affairs and/or to make specified decisions about personal welfare, including medical treatment.

The Enduring Powers of Attorney (Northern Ireland) Order 1987

This allows for the appointment of an attorney to make decisions regarding financial and property matters only (Enduring Power of Attorney). There is no specific legislation governing management of health and welfare of people without capacity in Northern Ireland, although the Bamford Review (see Chapter 42) has recommended this.

Mental health legislation in England and Wales

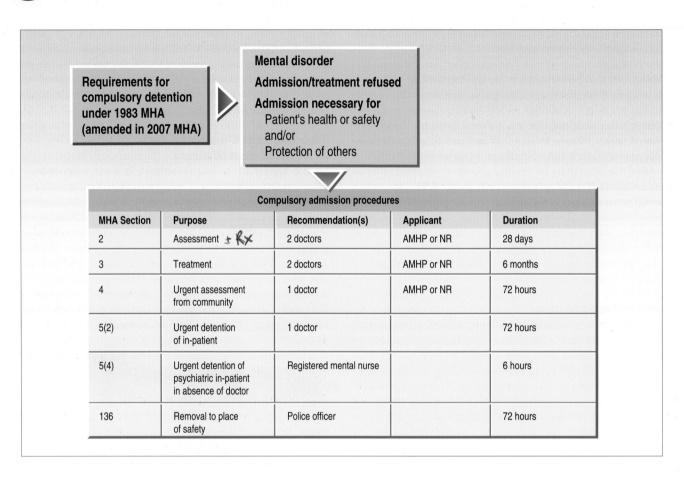

MHA Section	Purpose	Recommendation(s)	Applicant	Duration
2	Assessment + Rx	2 doctors	AMHP or NR	28 days
3	Treatment	2 doctors	AMHP or NR	6 months
4	Urgent assessment from community	1 doctor	AMHP or NR	72 hours
5(2)	Urgent detention of in-patient	1 doctor		72 hours
5(4)	Urgent detention of psychiatric in-patient in absence of doctor	Registered mental nurse		6 hours
136	Removal to place of safety	Police officer		72 hours

Introduction

The Mental Health Act (MHA) is primarily concerned with the care and treatment of patients compulsorily detained in hospital on medical recommendation or by court order. It is supervised by the Mental Health Act Commission (MHAC). The MHA 2007, due to be enacted in 2008, makes amendments to the 1983 Act.

Definitions

The MHA 1983 has four categories of mental disorder: *mental illness, mental impairment, severe mental impairment* and *psychopathic disorder* (a legal term comparable to antisocial personality disorder). The 2007 MHA amends this to a single category, *mental disorder* (MD), meaning any disorder or disability of the mind. This broader definition of mental disorder includes some people (e.g. those with personality disorders other than antisocial personality disorder) not covered by the 1983 Act. The MHA does not regard dependence on alcohol or drugs as evidence of MD. The 1983 Act excluded sexual deviancy (which would include paraphilias such as fetishism or paedophilia [Chapter 15]) as a reason for detention, but the 2007 Act does not.

Requirements for detention

Compulsory admission ('sectioning') requires that a patient is judged to have a MD of sufficient severity to warrant detention in hospital in the interests of his or her health and/or safety and/or for the protection of others.

There are additional criteria that must be met for patients to be detained under the longer-lasting sections (sections 3 and 37). In the 1983 MHA, patients can only be detained on these sections under the categories of *mental impairment* or *psychopathic disorder* to receive treatment that is likely to alleviate or prevent deterioration. In the 2007 Act, this condition is amended to a requirement that appropriate medical treatment is available to them; it adds that people cannot be detained due to learning disability alone unless this is associated with abnormally aggressive or seriously irresponsible conduct.

For treatment to continue beyond the first three months, the patient must either consent (and be attested competent to do so by a responsible clinician [RC]), or the treatment plan must be agreed necessary by an independent 'second opinion' psychiatrist nominated by the MHAC.

How 'sectioning' is carried out

Most hospital detentions are under section 2 or 3. Application for these sections under the 1983 Act is made by a social worker 'approved' under the MHA (ASW). The 2007 MHA extends this role (renamed the approved mental health professional [AMHP]), to other professionals, including nurses, psychologists and occupational therapists. Rarely, the nearest relative may make the application. Application is made on the recommendations of two doctors, one a specialist 'approved' under section 12 of the MHA. The other doctor must either be section 12-approved or have 'previous knowledge' of the patient (e.g. the patient's GP). For section 3, the ASW/AMHP has a duty to consult the nearest relative if possible; if the relative objects, the section cannot proceed unless the RC takes legal action to displace the relative.

MHA assessments are convened by the ASW/AMHP, often at the patient's home or in A&E. Two doctors and the ASW/AMHP assess the patient, and if they decide that he or she should be hospitalized and the patient refuses informal admission, arrange admission under section. The police may attend assessments if there are concerns that the patient will be violent or physically resist coming to hospital if detained. Where a patient lacks capacity to agree to an informal admission (e.g. due to dementia), he or she may still be admitted informally so long as the patient appears to assent and does not object. Such admission are subject to the provisions of the Mental Capacity Act 2005 (see Chapter 39).

Leave and discharge from section

Section 17 requires that patients on sections 2 and 3 can only be placed on leave subject to the RC's specific instructions.

Patients may be discharged from a section 2 or 3 before it expires at the discretion of the RC. Patients may appeal to a Mental Health Review Tribunal (MHRT) within 14 days for section 2 or at any time within the first six months and once during each subsequent period of renewal for section 3. MHRTs consist of a lawyer (president), psychiatrist and a lay member (for section 41 patients the president is a judge or Queen's Counsel). Patients may be granted legal aid and obtain an independent medical opinion. They may also appeal to hospital managers (community members who act as non-executive directors of a hospital) for discharge. Alternatively, the nearest relative may implement discharge, although they must give 72 hours' notice and can be barred in some circumstances by the RC. *Section 117* requires that a multidisciplinary meeting be convened to ensure adequate aftercare for any patient discharged from section 3.

Section 2, admission for assessment (or for assessment followed by medical treatment), lasts for 28 days.

Section 3, admission for treatment, lasts six months (and is renewable).

Section 4, emergency assessment, lasts 72 hours and is applied for by the ASW/AMHP or nearest relative. One doctor (preferably with previous knowledge of the patient) makes the recommendation on the grounds that admission (otherwise fulfilling section 2 requirements) is more urgent than section 2 procedures would allow.

Section 136 empowers a police officer who finds a person in a public place appearing to suffer from a MD to remove him or her to a 'place of safety' for assessment. It is valid for 72 hours.

Section 135, which lasts 72 hours, empowers a police officer or other authorized person acting on a magistrate's warrant to enter premises and remove to a place of safety a person who is believed to be suffering from a MD.

Section 5(2), for patients already in hospital (receiving any form of treatment), is valid for 72 hours and is on the recommendation of the doctor in charge of the case or his/her nominated deputy. Patients placed on section 5(2) must subsequently be assessed for section 2 or 3 or discharged from section 5(2), to become an informal patient.

Registered mental nurses (RMNs) may make the recommendation for *section 5(4)*, which allows urgent detention for up to six hours of a patient already receiving treatment for MD in hospital when a doctor is not able to attend immediately.

Community treatment

Guardianship (sections 7 and 8) is intended to ensure that adults with MD receive proper care and protection in the community. The guardian (usually an ASW/AMHP) is nominated by the local authority and is empowered to ensure that the individual resides at a specified place, attends specified places and times for treatment, education, training or occupation and allows specified people (e.g. ASW/AMHPs, doctors) access to their residence.

Supervised community treatment (SCT) is introduced in the 2007 MHA to replace the earlier *supervised discharge* order (section 25). Patients may be placed on a SCT following a period of detention in hospital under section 3 or 37 by application of the RC with agreement of AMHP. It requires that the patient make him- or herself available for medical examination. Patients may be recalled to hospital if: they require treatment on grounds of their health or safety which can only be given in hospital; they refuse to make themselves available for examination by the RC; or they do not comply with conditions of the SCT. This strengthens the provisions of the supervised discharge order, the only enforceable aspect of which is the power to convey the person to a place of safety or a place for treatment, and did not permit the person to be treated or detained in hospital for longer than required for an assessment to be carried out.

Sections relating to prisoners

Section 35, empowering a Crown or Magistrate's Court to remand an accused person to a specific hospital for a report, lasts for 28 days, is applied for at trial by defence or prosecution counsel or by the court, and requires written or oral evidence from one medical practitioner.

Section 36, empowering a Crown Court to remand an accused individual to hospital for treatment, is valid for 28 days and is based on two medical reports (one from an 'approved doctor'). Appropriate medical treatment must be available.

Section 37 empowers a Crown or Magistrate's Court to order hospital admission or the reception into guardianship of a person convicted of an imprisonable offence (except murder).

Section 41, a restriction order (by Crown Court only), is based on the oral evidence of one doctor and added to hospital orders. Restricted patients may not be given leave, transferred or discharged without the consent of the Home Secretary.

Treatment orders

Section 57 concerns treatment requiring both consent and a second opinion (e.g. psychosurgery, surgical implants of hormones).

Section 58 concerns treatment requiring consent or a second opinion (e.g. ECT, medications for longer than six months) (see Chapter 37 for ECT). Under *Section 62*, urgent life-saving treatment may be exempted from sections 57 and 58.

Requirements for compulsory detention under Mental Health (Care and Treatment) Scotland Act 2003	Mental disorder which significantly impairs decision-making ability of patient with respect to medical treatment *Admission necessary for:* Patient's health or safety and/or Protection of others

MHA order	Purpose	Location	Requirements	Duration
Emergency detention	Urgent assessment where arranging short-term detention under order would cause unacceptable delay	Hospital	One fully registered doctor with (where possible) consent of MHO	<72hrs
Short term detention	Assessment or treatment	Hospital	One AMP recommendation agreed by MHO	<28 days
Compulsory Treatment	Treatment (in community) requires certain place of residence or attendance for treatment	Hospital or community	Application by MHO, 2 AMP recommentations Decision by Mental Health Tribunal	<6 months

MHO = Mental Health Officer; AMP = Approved Mental Practitioner

The Mental Health (Care and Treatment) (Scotland) Act 2003 concerns the compulsory treatment of people with mental disorders living in Scotland. It amends the Criminal Procedure (Scotland) Act 1995 regarding the treatment of mentally disordered offenders. The Mental Welfare Commission is an independent body which monitors the operation of the Act and promotes best practice. It appoints designated medical practitioners when circumstances require a second medical opinion on compulsory treatment.

The 2003 Act gives people with a mental disorder a right to independent *advocacy*. Additionally, any adult can appoint a *named person* (if this is agreed in writing and witnessed) who has a right to be consulted and to appeal against the detention of the person they support. The Act also allows people to make *advance statements* about how they would wish to be treated if they become unable to express their views as a result of becoming mentally unwell. The Tribunal and doctors treating the person must take notice of an advance statement and inform the patient, the patient's named person and the Mental Welfare Commission in writing of the reasons if they do not follow it.

Compulsory orders

To be detained, a person must be suffering from a *mental disorder* (mental illness [including dementia], personality disorder or learning disability] which *significantly impairs* their decision-making with respect to medical treatment of the disorder; and would put their health, safety or welfare, or the safety of another, at significant risk if they were not detained. Detention must be deemed necessary. Significantly impaired decision-making ability is not the same as 'incapacity' under the Adults with Incapacity (Scotland) Act 2000 (see Chapter 39), but is a related concept. It refers to the specific capacity of an individual to make decisions about medical treatment for mental disorder, whereas the Adults with Incapacity (Scotland) Act 2000 covers a range of different capacities.

Emergency detention (<72 hours) may be certified by any fully registered doctor who should gain the consent of a *Mental Health Officer* (MHO; a social worker with additional training) if possible. Detention must be necessary for urgent assessment, while arranging assessment for a short-term detention certificate (see below) would involve undesirable delay. It is good practice to use the short-term detention order wherever possible.

Short-term detention (<28 days) is for assessment or treatment, with criteria similar to emergency detention. It is recommended by an *approved medical practitioner* (AMP) (a doctor with mental health expertise, usually a psychiatrist) and agreed by a MHO. The certificate may be cancelled by the responsible medical officer (RMO), Tribunal or the Mental Welfare Commission if the person no longer fulfils the criteria. The patient and their named person can ask the Mental Health Tribunal (see below) to review the case.

A *Compulsory Treatment Order* (CTO) requires that medical treatment is available which may prevent deterioration, or help treat any symptoms or effects of the mental disorder, and without which there would be a significant risk to the person or others. Medical treatment may include nursing care, psychological intervention, education and training in living skills. It lasts up to six months initially, can be extended for a further six months, and subsequently for 12 months at a time. It may be based in the hospital or the community. A community order may require the patient to receive medical treatment (but not by force), live at a certain address and attend certain services for treatment. The decision on whether to grant a CTO is made by the Mental Health Tribunal. Tribunals have three panel members: a lawyer, a doctor with experience in mental health and third person with other skills and experience. A MHO makes an application to the Tribunal, including two medical recommendations and a proposed care plan. Patients are given the opportunity to express their views if they wish to at the Tribunal.

If the Tribunal needs further information before making a final decision or the patient, or their solicitor needs more time to prepare their case, the Tribunal may make an *interim (temporary) CTO* (<28 days), which can be renewed once only. A CTO can be ended by the RMO, Tribunal or the Mental Welfare Commission. The patient or their named person has the right to appeal against decisions made by the Tribunal.

Nurses' holding power – an appropriately qualified nurse can hold a hospital patient who has been receiving treatment on a voluntary basis for up to two hours to allow a doctor to assess the patient. This can be extended by another one hour once the doctor arrives.

Removal to place of safety – the police can take a person from a public place to a place of safety for <24 hours if they appear to have a mental disorder and be in need of care and treatment, for assessment.

Mental health law relating to prisoners

The court can make an assessment and treatment orders at any stage of the criminal justice process prior to sentencing. An *assessment order* allows a person to be detained in hospital for up to 28 days. *Interim compulsion orders* provide for a longer period of assessment (up to a year, with renewal every 12 weeks). A *treatment order* allows for a person with a mental disorder to receive required care and treatment in hospital; it ceases at the end of the period for which the person is on remand or is committed.

Compulsion order

This is similar to a CTO (see above), except the requirement for significantly impaired decision-making ability with regard to treatment does not apply. Where a person presents a serious risk to the public, it may be combined with a *restriction order*, meaning any change in the legal status of the patient must be referred to the Scottish Ministers and subsequently the Tribunal.

Assessment orders require evidence from one medical practitioner; interim compulsion, compulsion and treatment orders from two medical practitioners, one an AMP. A compulsion order also requires a report from the designated MHO.

Transfer for treatment directions

This order, made by Scottish ministers, permits the transfer of prisoners to hospital for treatment of a mental disorder. It requires the evidence of two medical practitioners (one an AMP). It ceases upon the expiry of the person's sentence.

The court may detain a person who has been acquitted of an offence but may require admission to hospital for treatment of a mental disorder in a place of safety for < six hours so a medical examination can be carried out.

Medical treatment

Urgent treatment that is not associated with significant risks or irreversible consequences may be given without consent to save the patient's life, to alleviate serious suffering on the part of the patient or to prevent violent or dangerous behaviour. Where a detained patient does not or cannot consent to drug treatment, it must be authorized by an independent medical practitioner to continue beyond two months.

Electroconvulsive therapy (ECT) may only be given to a patient if he or she can and does consent, or is incapable of consenting and the treatment is authorized by an independent medical practitioner. ECT cannot be given to a patient who has capacity and refuses the treatment, even in an emergency. Neurosurgery for mental disorder can only be carried out after an independent medical practitioner gives an opinion that it will be beneficial to the patient, and two lay people appointed by the Commission have certified that the person consents, or does not object if they are incapable of giving consent. Where the person is incapable of consenting, the Court of Session must also give approval.

Requirements for compulsory detention under 1986 Mental Health (Northern Ireland) Order	Mental disorder Admission/treatment refused Admission necessary to prevent substantial risk of serious physical harm to patient or other

To detain a voluntary inpatient who is refusing treatment or to stay in hospital:
Doctor (usually junior doctor) completes form 5/5a then proceeds as below.

All patients initially detained for up to 14 days. Requires:
- Recommendation of one doctor (who completes form 3)
- Application by ASW

To extend detention, consultant must complete:
- Form 8 (in first 7 days)
- Form 9 (in second 7 days)
- Form 10 (detention for 6 months)

The 1986 Mental Health (Northern Ireland) Order makes provision for the detention, guardianship, care and treatment of patients. Its use is monitored by the Mental Health Commission of Northern Ireland. The Bamford Review (2002–6) suggested changes to legislation similar to those that have recently been implemented in Scotland, England and Wales (see Chapters 40 and 41).

Criteria for detention

The definition of mental disorder comprises mental illness, mental handicap, severe mental handicap and severe mental impairment. Mental illness is defined as a 'state of mind which affects a person's thinking, perceiving, emotion or judgement to the extent that he requires care or medical treatment in his own interests or the interests of other persons'. The order cannot be used for the compulsory treatment of addictions, personality disorders (unlike the legislation in England, Wales or Scotland) or sexual deviancy, unless the above criteria are also met. Persons may be detained only if they are suffering from a mental disorder of a nature or degree that warrants detention in hospital for assessment (or for assessment followed by medical treatment); and failure to detain the patient would create a substantial likelihood of serious physical harm to the patient or to others. Criteria for likelihood of serious physical harm are that the patient has inflicted, or threatened or attempted to inflict, serious physical harm on themselves; the patient's judgement is so affected that they are, or would soon be, unable to protect themselves against serious physical harm and that reasonable provision for their protection is not available in the community; or that other persons have reasonable fear they may suffer serious physical harm due to violent or other behaviour of the person.

Compulsory admission to hospital

Article 4 permits a patient to be compulsorily admitted and detained in hospital for assessment on the application of the nearest relative or an approved social worker (ASW). This application must be supported by the recommendation of one doctor (who completes a Form 3) and the doctor and ASW must have seen the patient in the two days preceding the application. The doctor should (if possible) know the patient and not be (except in cases of urgent necessity) on the staff of the receiving hospital. In practice, the doctor is usually the patient's GP. All detained patients are initially admitted for a period of assessment of up to 14 days.

A doctor must assess the patient immediately after admission to hospital (and complete a Form 7). If the admitting doctor is not a consultant, the patient must be seen by a consultant within 48 hours of admission. If the patient is further detained, he or she will be seen again by a consultant (who will complete a Form 8 and Form 9 for these respective time periods) within the first and second seven-day periods of the admission. The consultant may then complete a Form 10, which allows detention for treatment (six months in the first instance). This may be extended for a second six-month period (Form 11), and thereafter for periods of one year (for which a Form 12 must be signed by two consultants).

Police powers

A police officer may remove from a public place an individual who appears to be suffering from a mental disorder and in need of immediate care and control, and take the person to a place of safety (usually a police station), where they must be seen by a doctor and ASW. If the person is not in a public place and access to the property is denied, a warrant to enter the premises may be obtained (Article 129) by an ASW, another officer of the Health and Social Services Trust or a police officer from a Justice of the Peace. If the police officer has to enter the premises, by force or otherwise, he or she must be accompanied by a medical practitioner (usually a GP) who will administer medical treatment if required. The person may then be transferred to a place of safety.

Informal hospital patients

A patient who has been admitted informally and subsequently wants to leave or refuse treatment may be detained if appropriate by completion of a Form 5 or 5a (for psychiatric and general hospital patients respectively), usually by a junior doctor. The patient's own GP (or another practitioner who has previous knowledge of the patient) must then attend the hospital to complete a medical recommendation (Form 3), and an ASW or nearest relative must make an application, after which matters proceed as for other detained patients. A doctor on the staff of the hospital in which it is intended that the assessment should be carried out cannot give the recommendation except in a case of urgent necessity.

Guardianship

A guardianship order may require the patient to: reside at a certain place, attend at specified places and times for the purpose of medical treatment, occupation, education or training, and allow any specified doctor, ASW or other person access to their residence. The order lasts for six months initially, and may then be renewed for a further six months and yearly thereafter.

Persons aged 16 or over may be subject to a guardianship order if they are found to be suffering from mental illness or severe mental handicap and it is deemed necessary in the interests of their welfare. The application may be made by an ASW or the patient's nearest relative, who must have personally seen the patient within 14 days of the application, and be supported by two medical recommendations. The ASW should consult the nearest relative if possible. If the nearest relative objects, involvement of a second ASW is required. The nominated guardian is normally a social worker.

Patients involved in criminal proceedings

Courts may remand an unsentenced prisoner to hospital for two weeks (Article 42) for the preparation of reports or for treatment (Article 43).

A remand under Article 42 can be made on the basis of one medical opinion – the oral evidence of a Part II-approved doctor (in practice, a consultant). Article 42 does not allow treatment without the patient's consent, or granting of temporary leave from the hospital by the Responsible Medical Officer.

The court may make a hospital or guardianship order or hospital order with restriction when sentencing a prisoner (Article 44) on receipt of evidence from two medical practitioners, one of whom must be Part II-approved and give oral evidence. An interim hospital order allows admission to hospital before the court makes a hospital order.

A person serving a sentence of imprisonment may be transferred to hospital for treatment after two written reports have been provided to the Secretary of State (Article 53). Article 53 requires 'that the person is suffering from mental illness or severe mental impairment'.

Appeal

The Mental Health Review Tribunal hears appeals against detention in hospital or guardianship orders. It consists of a legal member who is the president, a medical member and a lay member. Referral to the Tribunal may be by the patient or nearest relative and the Hospital Trust must refer any patient who has been detained for two years without a tribunal hearing. Under the 1986 Order, the patient needed to prove that he or she should be released. This was found to be incompatible with the European Convention on Human Rights. The Mental Health (Amendment) (Northern Ireland) Order 2004 has therefore amended the 1986 Order to shift the burden of proof to the Health and Social Services Trust to demonstrate that a patient should *not* be discharged.

Consent to treatment

This legislation is similar to the 1983 Mental Health Act (England and Wales) provision (Chapter 40). *Article 63* states that patients may not receive neurosurgery for mental disorder unless they consent and the treatment is recommended in a second opinion from an independent doctor. These safeguards apply to both detained patients and voluntary patients. *Article 64* covers other serious forms of treatment and requires either the patient's consent or a second medical opinion (e.g. for ECT). These requirements apply only to detained patients. *Article 68* deals with cases requiring urgent treatment required for certain specified emergencies (e.g. ECT) which may be given without the patient's consent or a second medical opinion.

OSCEs

Increased
  Fairness
  Reliability
Emphasis on communication skills
VITAL to stick to
  Task(s)
  Time
    5–10 minutes on each
  Note role
    GP
    Psychiatrist
  Do NOT repeat task verbatim
  AVOID technical language
  Ensure actor (patient) has chance to speak
Typical 'tasks' include
  Assessing suicide risk
  Eliciting an aspect of the psychiatric history
  Eliciting an aspect of the mental state
  Talking to a relative
  Explaining a diagnosis
  Assessing a patient who arrives smelling of alcohol
  Talking to a patient who has cut him/herself
  Dealing with any specified psychiatric emergency

General principles

Put patient at ease
  Greet and introduce
  Explain your purpose
Current symptoms may be absent
Use open questions
Reflect and clarify
Acknowledge distress
Observe
  Behaviour
    Obvious physical signs
Say goodbye and express thanks

Short cases

Stick to task
Be systematic
Do not repeat task verbatim
  to patient
Be prepared to
  Summarize
  Reach clear conclusions

Long cases

Aims
  (Differential) diagnosis
  Aetiology
  Management plan
  Prognosis
Organize interview and summarize
  systematically
  History (see Chapter 1)
  Mental state (see Chapter 1)
  Physical examination as
    appropriate

Introduction

Objective Structured Clinical Examinations (OSCEs) are now used in most UK medical schools to assess clinical aspects of psychiatry. In this chapter we outline some typical types of OSCE station, with some prac-tice tips. Short and long cases are still occasionally used for assessment so these are also discussed. General interviewing tips are:

• Always start with a polite introduction and thank the patient at the end. Ask the patient what he or she wants to be called.

• Use a mix of open questions to start off (to which a longer descriptive answer is expected) and closed questions (yes/no answers).

• Listen to the patient and ask follow-up questions to clarify any points that are not clear.

• Use language which is understandable to people without a medical degree.

• Acknowledge any distress a patient shows (e.g. 'I'm sorry this is upsetting').

• It is often helpful to summarize to the patient what has been said, par-ticularly if you are unsure what was meant.

Observed structured clinical examinations

An OSCE examination consists of several (usually 8–12) stations with a standard and relatively short time (5–10 minutes) spent on each. Stick-ing to task and time is therefore vital. Remember that the marking system is standardized, and that stations are distributed across the main areas that you should cover. A good revision technique is to write some OSCE stations yourselves, preferably in a revision group, and devise your own marking sheet (see our examples in the self-assessment section of this book).

Read the question carefully, and re-read it, taking 10–15 seconds at the beginning (longer than it sounds!) to make sure you are clear what the task is and to marshal your thoughts about how to begin. Take note of your role (GP, psychiatrist), and introduce yourself as this. Also take note of what the patient or relative is expecting. For example, if you have been asked to assess alcohol use or memory in someone who has come about a different matter, saying 'I understand you're here about your alcohol/memory problem' could get you off to a bad start. Don't waste time discussing things that are not relevant to the task. If the ques-tion says 'Assess this man's current risk of suicide', you will get marks for asking about his current thoughts, plans and intentions, so don't let the conversation drift to a prolonged discussion of an overdose years ago. Do not repeat the task verbatim to the patient (e.g. do not say 'I have been asked to ask you if you have any abnormal beliefs' or 'I am going to ask you about suicide').

Here are some typical tasks requested in OSCE stations and tips on how to address them:

Giving information to a patient or relative, about a diagnosis, treatment or prognosis

You will not be expected to take a history on such stations unless the question specifically tells you to do so.

Practise succinctly explaining the main psychiatric diagnoses (e.g. schizophrenia, bipolar affective disorder, depression, dementia); try to avoid technical language, or explain any terms you use (e.g. 'tests of kidney function', not 'U&Es').

Ensure that you first check what the patient/carer knows and a little bit about their particular condition. They want to know about their own illness, not about the condition generally.

Ask if there are things they particularly want to know, and after giving your explanation, check if that answers their questions.

Ensure the actor has a chance to speak; it is not a mini-lecture and people can only take a few pieces of information on board at a time.

At the end, explain how they can get in touch with someone (care coordinator, GP, etc.) in the future and offer to send them leaflets, or refer them to appropriate internet sites (e.g. MIND, Alzheimer's Society) to show you know that they will not remember everything.

Assessing suicide risk

This is a very common station, so well worth practising. If you are asked to assess someone's level of suicide risk after a recent attempt, make sure you elicit the key factors in the attempt (were they alone? was it planned? perceived lethality, etc.) as well as how they feel about it now (thoughts, plans, intent). If asked to assess suicide risk, the number of past attempts and family history are relevant factors, but don't get bogged down in the past history at the expense of current mental state and the recent attempt.

Eliciting an aspect of the psychiatric history

This will be in a very focused area, such as taking an alcohol or illicit substance use history.

Eliciting an aspect of the mental state

Again this will be in a focused area. Make sure you do not drift into taking a history. For example, if asked to elicit symptoms of depression, ask about current mood, ability to enjoy life, energy levels, negative cognitions (guilt, hopelessness), biological symptoms, etc. Don't ask when they first became depressed.

Video stations

You may be asked to assess a mental state from a video. A good way to practise this is to try to write a mental state for a patient you have seen in a ward round and ask for feedback, or compare with a recent clerking. Make sure you write something for every section, even if there is no abnormality you can see, e.g. 'cognition grossly normal' or 'no perceptual abnormality detected'. Watch for physical signs (e.g. tremor or other extrapyramidal signs, tics, exophthalmos, evidence of liver disease, tattoos, scars, needle marks, obviously over-/underweight, clothes too big) and abnormal or indicative behaviours, such as crying or poor eye contact.

Other stations

You may be asked to discuss a drug chart or section paper (so make sure you have seen and discussed some during your clinical attachment).

Short and long cases

These are now employed less frequently in assessments.

Short cases

This part of the exam can consist of between one and four cases. You may be asked to take a particular part of the history (e.g. 'This patient has a drinking problem; please take an alcohol history') or examine a particular aspect of the mental state (e.g. 'Does this patient have Schneiderian first-rank symptoms?'). You may also be asked to perform a full mental state examination or a full cognitive examination. As for OSCEs, make sure you have fully understood the task(s) assigned to you. Introduce yourself and the examiner(s), explain what you have been asked to do (reiterating that this is an exam rather than a clinical situation) and be seen to put the patient at ease. It is equally important to be seen to be systematic. You are likely to be asked what you elicited and concluded at the end.

Long cases

This involves interviewing a patient at length (usually 45–60 minutes) uninterrupted (and unobserved) with the aim of reaching a diagnosis or differential diagnosis, as well as discussing aetiology, principles of medical and psychosocial management and prognosis. You will be given a few minutes after the patient has left to collect and organize your findings for the presentation. Be systematic during both the interview and the summarizing process, using headings for the history and mental state examination as outlined in Chapters 1 and 2. Clarify the patient's current status (in/outpatient, detained/informal) and any recent or significant life-events (see Chapter 10). Remember that psychiatric patients often have significant physical comorbidity and that non-psychiatric examiners may be particularly interested in these aspects. Always leave enough time for a brief but appropriate physical examination. You should try to summarize the key features of the case at the end of your presentation. Attempt a diagnosis using one of the classificatory systems outlined in Chapter 3. If you have had any difficulty in taking the history (some patients are suspicious or unforthcoming) it is important to say so and to remember that this should not be to your disadvantage. You may be asked to repeat some of the interview in front of the examiner(s), in which case apply the principles discussed for short cases.

Sample OSCE stations

Station 1

Candidate instructions

You are a GP. A woman who was recently diagnosed with bipolar affective disorder has come to see you and wants to discuss her diagnosis. She has some questions about her disorder and her medication on discharge (lithium carbonate).
Please answer her questions. You do not need to take a history.

Sample interview

Candidate: Hello, my name is Dr Smith. How can I help you?

Patient: *I just wanted some information really about the diagnosis I was given at the hospital. They told me I had bipolar affective disorder. What does that mean?*

Candidate: Sure. Can I ask what you've been told so far about that, so I don't repeat what you already know?

Patient: *Not much really, that it's a mental illness and that it's caused by an imbalance or something.*

Candidate: Bipolar affective disorder is a mental illness that affects mood. People with bipolar disorder have episodes, called manic episodes, when their mood and self-esteem are increased. They often have a decreased need for sleep, talk more and start to believe that they have special abilities or gifts. It can be dangerous as sometimes people act very impulsively or take risks they would not normally take. They also have times of feeling very depressed. Between these two types of illness (depression and manic episodes) people with bipolar feel well and are able to go about life as normal. Does that make sense?

Patient: *Yes, I think so. It's a lot to remember all at once.*

Candidate: Sure. We have some leaflets in the surgery with some more information about bipolar affective disorder which I could give you, if you would find that helpful.

Patient: *Thanks, that would be good. Also, I have been told I will need to have blood tests while I am taking lithium. What are they for?*

Candidate: As with all drugs, lithium can have side-effects. It can cause kidney or thyroid problems. Therefore, we monitor thyroid and kidney function through blood tests, at least once a year. That way, if problems do occur we can pick them up and manage them. Lithium works best when it is above a certain concentration in the blood stream, but if levels become too high, it can be dangerous. Therefore, we also monitor the lithium levels.

Patient: *I see. What should I do if I want to stop my medication?*

Candidate: It is important to talk to me or another doctor if you want to stop your medication. Depending on your reasons for wanting to stop, we could consider a different medication. I would strongly suggest you do take medication as it considerably decreases your chances of having another episode, and the severity of the illness if you do have one. If you do decide you want to stop your medication, it is safer to do this gradually and this could also be discussed with your doctor at the time.

Patient: *If I tell you I have stopped my medication will I be sectioned again?*

Candidate: You are receiving treatment voluntarily now and it is your right to stop if you want to. You would not be sectioned just because you stopped your medication, but it would increase your chances of becoming unwell again. A Mental Health Act assessment may be arranged if you were unwell, we were seriously concerned about your mental health or your safety and you were refusing treatment for your illness.
Do you have any questions about that?

Patient: *On another subject, I have been wondering what I should do about the medication if I want to get pregnant?*

Candidate: My advice would be to come and talk to me or another doctor before you started trying to conceive. That way you could discuss with us the risks and benefits of taking medication for your illness during pregnancy. Lithium, in common with some other medications, is associated with an increased risk of harm to your unborn child, and it might be appropriate to change to another drug. It is also important for you and your unborn child that you stay well during and after your pregnancy, so as I said, the risks and concerns about medication would need to be considered carefully at that time.
Has that answered your question?

Patient: *Yes, thanks.*

Station 2

Candidate instructions

You are a junior psychiatrist working in a Community Mental Health Team. One of the social workers, Tom, asks you to see a 28-year-old woman with a diagnosis of depression. She has a three-year-old son, Charlie, who is seen by a child and family social worker regularly. Assess the risk of self-harm and any risk to the child. You have read the past psychiatric history and other background information, so focus on the current situation.

Sample interview

Candidate (After polite introduction): Tom has told me that you are very unhappy at the moment. Is that right?

Patient: *Yes, I feel really awful.*

Candidate: Have things got so bad that you feel you don't want to live any more?

Patient: *(Nods, despondently).*

Candidate: Are you thinking about harming yourself?

Patient: *I have thought about it.*

Candidate: What have you thought of doing?

Patient: *Taking an overdose.*

Candidate: What's the nearest you've got recently to actually doing that?

Patient: *Not that near yet, really.*

Candidate: Have you thought what tablets you would take?

Patient: *I've got lots of paracetamol at home. I've thought of taking them.*

Candidate: And does it feel at the moment like you would do that?

Patient: *Probably not, no. I don't think I actually would.*

Candidate: How are you managing to stop yourself from taking them?

Patient: *I think about my husband and Charlie and how upset they would be. I couldn't let Charlie grow up without a mother.*

Candidate: If the thoughts returned, is there anyone you might feel able to talk to?

Patient: *My parents, or maybe the crisis team. They gave me their number and said I could call them if I felt like that.*

Candidate: And do you think you would call them if you felt close to harming yourself.

Patient: *Yes, I would.*

Candidate: Is it difficult looking after Charlie while you are feeling so distressed?

Patient: *It can be, but I have lots of help. My husband works from home, so he has been around most of the time, and if he has to go into the office, my mother has been coming round to help me.*

Candidate: Have you ever had thought that you might hurt Charlie in some way?

Patient: *No, never. He's my reason to live.*

[End of patient interview]

Examiner: How do you think this lady's risk should be managed?

Candidate: She should be referred to the crisis team. They can monitor the risk and consider inpatient treatment if the situation worsens.

Examiner: Do you think it is safe for Charlie to stay at home while she is unwell?

Candidate: Yes.

EMQs

1. Treatment in psychiatry
(a) Antipsychotic medication
(b) Benzodiazepine
(c) CBT alone
(d) ECT
(e) Family therapy
(f) Mood stabilizer
(g) Psychodynamic psychotherapy
(h) SSRI and CBT
(i) SSRI only
(j) Vagal nerve stimulation

Which of these would be the most appropriate treatment for the following situations? Choose one option. Each option may be used once, more than once, or not at all.

1. A 64-year-old man has been severely depressed for several months; his condition is deteriorating despite treatment with antidepressants. He is very distressed, suicidal and is refusing to eat.
2. A 31-year-old mother of a two-month-old baby asks her GP for help. Her GP diagnoses mild depressive disorder.
3. A 28-year-old man presents with severe obsessive compulsive disorder. He is no longer able to go to work as it takes him several hours to get dressed every morning due to compulsive rituals.
4. A 34-year-old woman seeks help from her GP. She is concerned that she has problems in intimate relationships due to sexual abuse that she experienced as a child. She feels this is making her very anxious.
5. An 11-year-old boy is brought to the child psychiatry clinic by his mother. She is concerned that he is very distressed and has started to misbehave at school as a result of family difficulties. His father recently moved back home after a period of marital separation.

2. Epidemiology in psychiatry
(a) 1%
(b) 5%
(c) 10%
(d) 20%
(e) 25%
(f) 40%
(g) 50%
(h) 60%
(i) 70%

Which of these percentages best estimates the following? Choose one option. Each option may be used once, more than once or not at all.

1. The lifetime prevalence of bipolar I disorder.
2. Approximate risk of the identical twin of a person with schizophrenia developing the same disorder.
3. Reported suicide rate among people with schizophrenia.
4. Percentage of the population who experience mental health problems at one time.
5. Percentage of men in the UK who are alcohol-dependent.
6. Percentage of UK deaths recorded as suicide.
7. The prevalence of dementia among people aged over 65.

3. Psychiatry and the law
(a) Mental Health Act (MHA), section 2
(b) MHA, section 3
(c) MHA, section 5(2)
(d) MHA, section 5(4)
(e) MHA, section 17
(f) MHA, section 37
(g) MHA, section 58
(h) MHA, section 117
(i) MHA, section 135
(j) MHA, section 136
(k) Mental Capacity Act

Which Act, or section, is most appropriate to use in these situations? Choose one option. Each option may be used once, more than once or not at all.

1. A 28-year-old man was admitted to an orthopaedic ward after jumping off a motorway bridge in a suicide attempt. He remains depressed and shortly after telling a student nurse he wanted to try again he asks to self-discharge. The nurses contact you, the FY2 doctor, to ask your advice.
2. Police officers are concerned about a woman acting bizarrely in a public place. They think she needs a psychiatric assessment.
3. You are called to assess an 83-year-old woman with dementia on a medical ward who is refusing potentially life-saving intravenous antibiotics for treatment of cellulitis. When you see her she thinks she is in her lunch club and does not seem able to understand why she needs treatment. Her daughter is asking the medics to go ahead and treat her.
4. You assess a man who was brought to A&E by his wife. He has threatened to set fire to next door's house as he believes MI5 are using it as a monitoring station; he has no psychiatric history. He wants to go home.
5. A consultant psychiatrist treating a man for a psychotic episode under section 3 of the MHA wants to send him home on leave for a few hours.
6. A 28-year-old woman was arrested after attacking a passer-by, who she believed was possessed by a demon that was trying to kill her. The courts find her guilty of grievous bodily harm and accept the recommendations of a psychiatric report that she should be detained in psychiatric hospital for treatment of a psychotic disorder.
7. You see a 45-year-old woman in psychiatric outpatients and diagnose her with a psychotic episode. Being section 12-approved, you complete a recommendation for a section 2. Unfortunately, while you are awaiting the arrival of the Approved Social Worker (ASW) and second doctor she leaves and returns

home. When the ASW and doctor go to see her at her home she refuses to let them in.

4. Substance misuse
(a) Alcohol
(b) Amphetamines
(c) Benzodiazepines
(d) Cannabis
(e) Cocaine
(f) Ecstasy (MDMA)
(g) Heroin
(h) *Khat*
(i) LSD
(j) Phencyclidine
(k) Solvents

To which drug do these statements most apply? Choose one option. Each option may be used once, more than once or not at all.

1. Overdose of this drug is treated with naloxone.
2. There is good evidence that people using this drug between the ages of 11 and 15 are more likely to develop schizophrenia in adult life.
3. A red rash around the mouth is a common sign of abuse.
4. Deaths from hyponatraemia caused by drinking too much water after taking this drug have been reported.
5. The drug that most commonly causes dementia.
6. Addiction is frequently iatrogenic.
7. Euphoria is frequently followed by a period of depression which is termed 'the crash'.

5. Mental state
(a) Compulsion
(b) Delusion
(c) Depersonalization
(d) Derealization
(e) Hallucination
(f) Illusion
(g) Obsession
(h) Overvalued idea
(i) Pseudo-hallucination
(j) Rumination

What psychiatric sign is being described in these examples? Choose one option. Each option may be used once, more than once or not at all.

1. A 28-year-old woman is unable to resist the urge to wash her hands repeatedly.
2. A man describes hearing the voice of his dead father 'from inside my head'.
3. A woman complains that she feels she is cut off from the world 'as if by a pane of glass'.
4. An anxious man continually reviews the events leading to the loss of his job and is driving his wife to distraction.
5. A student walking home at night misperceives a tree as a man about to jump out at her.
6. A man is becoming increasingly troubled that his neighbours are following him. He sees them out so often it feels like 'more than

just a coincidence'. He can, however, entertain the possibility he might be wrong about this, although he thinks it more likely that he is right.
7. A man has stopped using the train because every time he stands on a platform he feels an irresistible urge to jump in front of a train.

6. Delusions
(a) Capgras' syndrome
(b) Delusional perception
(c) Ekbom's syndrome
(d) Erotomanic delusions
(e) *Folie à deux*
(f) Fregoli's syndrome
(g) Grandiose delusion
(h) Nihilistic delusion
(i) Persecutory delusion
(j) Somatic passivity

Which delusion is being described in these examples? Choose one option. Each option may be used once, more than once or not at all.

1. A man hit his mother with a heavy saucepan because he believed she had been replaced by a robot of identical appearance. He explains he was trying to disable the robot to 'get my mother back'.
2. A woman believes she can feel her blood temperature rising and that it must be being controlled using lasers by an outside force.
3. A woman applies for transfer to another council house because she describes being 'plagued by ants' that are crawling over her. When the psychiatrist visits, she has many matchboxes and other receptacles lined up in which she has 'trapped them as evidence'. They appear to be empty.
4. An 84-year-old woman and her middle-aged learning disabled son are refusing to pay their rent as they believe the council are winding the meter on remotely to extract more money from them.
5. A 34-year-old woman is detained by police for causing a public nuisance. She believes she has been invested with special healing powers, and that God has told her she is the next Messiah.
6. A man with depression erroneously believes he has lost all his possessions and his house has been destroyed.
7. A man fled the country after seeing a bunch of flowers by the side of the road. He was convinced this was a sign left for him by the FBI that they wanted him dead.

7. Psychiatric treatment
(a) Atypical antipsychotic
(b) Barbiturate
(c) Benzodiazepine
(d) Cholinesterase inhibitor
(e) Electroconvulsive therapy
(f) Monoamine oxidase inhibitor
(g) Mood stabilizer
(h) Selective serotonin reuptake inhibitor
(i) Serotonin and noradrenalin reuptake inhibitor
(j) Tricyclic antidepressant
(k) Typical antipsychotic

Which treatment most fits these descriptions? Choose one option. Each option may be used once, more than once or not at all.

1. The most frequently prescribed class of antidepressant.
2. Commonly used for short-term symptomatic treatment of anxiety and insomnia.
3. Class of drug that includes donepezil.
4. Class of drug most associated with extrapyramidal side-effects.
5. Consuming pickled herring while taking this class of drug could cause a dangerous rise in blood pressure.
6. Treatment most associated with weight gain and type II diabetes mellitus.
7. Cannot be prescribed to patients detained under section 3 without consent or the recommendation of a second doctor.
8. Class of drug that includes venlafaxine.

8. Cognitive impairment
   (a) Alcohol-related dementia
   (b) Alzheimer's disease
   (c) Creutzfeldt-Jakob disease
   (d) Frontotemporal dementia
   (e) Huntington's disease
   (f) Lewy body dementia
   (g) Normal pressure hydrocephalus
   (h) Vascular dementia

These disorders are all associated with cognitive decline. Which is being described in these examples? Choose one option. Each option may be used once, more than once or not at all.

1. Urinary incontinence typically occurs early in this illness.
2. Early personality changes are characteristic of this illness.
3. People with the E4 allele of apolipoprotein are at increased risk of this disorder.
4. People with this disorder are usually extremely sensitive to the side-effects of antipsychotic medication.
5. This disorder is often associated with stepwise rather than gradual deterioration.
6. A hereditary disorder that typically begins between the ages of 30 and 45.
7. Myoclonic jerks are characteristic.

9. Personality disorders
   (a) Anankastic
   (b) Avoidant
   (c) Dependent
   (d) Dissocial
   (e) Borderline
   (f) Histrionic
   (g) Paranoid
   (h) Schizoid
   (i) Schizotypal

Which personality disorders are described below? Choose one option. Each option may be used once, more than once or not at all.

1. A middle-aged man is referred by Social Services. He has made repeated complaints about his neighbours and the condition of his council house. He also has a number of tribunals with his previous employer outstanding. When seen he does not exhibit any psychotic symptoms. He describes himself as having been persistently picked on throughout his life and says he has learnt 'to fight back through the law'. He thinks the referral to psychiatric services might be an attempt by Social Services to discredit his evidence. He has lived alone since his marriage ended; his persistent fears that his wife was being unfaithful, which proved unfounded, contributed to the ending of the relationship.
2. A 72-year-old woman has been persistently unable to cope with life since the death of her husband ten years ago. Throughout her life she has always hated being alone, but it is only in the last decade that she has not had someone always with her. She lived with her parents for the first 25 years of her life and then with her husband. She recalls that she was always by her mother's side and then always by her husband's side. Her husband made all the decisions and she always went along with these, even if she did not agree as she did not like upsetting him. She is fit and well, but is asking to move to a nursing home where she can be looked after.
3. A 28-year-old woman presents to A&E after slashing her wrists. She has self-harmed on over 100 previous occasions. On two of these she recalled wanting to die, otherwise she cut herself to relieve tension. She was sexually abused by her father as a child and feels self-harm is her way of coping with her feelings about this.
4. A personality disorder that is more common among those with relatives who have schizophrenia.
5. The personality disorder that is most prevalent among male prisoners.
6. The personality disorder for which dialectical behavioural therapy was developed.
7. Social skills training may be particularly helpful in alleviating high levels of social anxiety in people with this disorder.

10. Child and adolescent psychiatry
   (a) Anorexia nervosa
   (b) Attention deficit hyperactivity disorder
   (c) Autism
   (d) Conduct disorder
   (e) Depression
   (f) Generalized anxiety
   (g) Personality disorder
   (h) Schizophrenia
   (i) School refusal
   (j) Simple phobia

Among children and adolescents, of which disorders are these statements true? Choose one option. Each option may be used once, more than once or not at all.

1. Although associated with psychiatric morbidity, this is not an actual psychiatric diagnosis.
2. Associated with antisocial personality disorder in later life.
3. This diagnosis should not be made in childhood or adolescence.
4. Prevalence is particularly high in ballet schools.
5. This disorder can be treated with methylphenidate.
6. This disorder usually manifests by the age of three years.
7. Common in young children and usually not clinically significant.

Case studies and questions

Case 1

An 84-year-old woman is admitted to an acute medical ward where you are working as a psychiatric liaison doctor. She lives alone. According to her neighbour she remained active until a few days ago doing voluntary work for the League of Friends; she has some problems with her breathing. He recalls she was in hospital with a chest infection last year, but he has never noticed her having any problems with her memory or any abnormal thoughts. She was admitted with confusion, after being found on the floor by paramedics called by concerned neighbours who had not seen her for days. The patient tells you she was beaten up by the secret service who took her to a police station. She believes the secret police followed her home due to connections that her dead husband had with a foreign police force. She is irritable and has at times asked to go home as she believes she is still in the police station and has spent enough time there. She describes seeing many police officers sitting around drinking tea. Her speech is difficult to follow. She scores poorly on cognitive testing, most of which she is unable to complete due to poor concentration. The nurses tell you she was quite lucid earlier that day and they thought she had improved, but her confusion has now worsened.

1 *What psychotic symptoms are present?*
2 *What is the most likely diagnosis, and what aspects of the history lead you this conclusion?*
3 *List five common causes of an acute confusional state.*
4 *What advice would you give regarding non-drug treatment of her confusion?*
5 *What advice would you give regarding drug treatment of her confusion?*
6 *What should happen if she asks to leave the ward?*

Case 2

While working as a psychiatric liaison doctor, you are called to the orthopaedic ward to assess John Baker, an unemployed 44-year-old with no previous psychiatric history who jumped off a motorway bridge three months ago in an apparent suicide attempt. He is physically well and about to be discharged. He was diagnosed with HIV some years ago. His partner recently died from AIDS. He tells you he tried to kill himself because he did not want to go on without her and still does not. The nurses report he has been quiet, withdrawn and tearful. They are concerned that he has been eating and drinking little. On examination he reports feeling worthless and says that there is no point to his life, as his partner was his only friend. He wants to die.

1 *What is the likely diagnosis?*
2 *What is the current suicide risk?*

He says that he recently saw his partner walk into the ward kitchen and momentarily felt comforted, although now he is worried that he is 'seeing things'.

3 *What would you advise him about his concerns regarding seeing his dead partner?*
4 *What treatment would you advise in this case?*

You decide to prescribe mirtazapine, but Mr Baker is reluctant to take it as he sees no point and believes nothing will help him. He has been told that he is fit for discharge and plans to go home the next day. You are concerned about this, place him on a section 5(2) and call the Approved Social Worker to arrange a Mental Health Act assessment.

5 *Under which section of the Mental Health Act would he be placed if he was detained at the assessment and why?*
6 *He makes good progress on the ward, and the consultant asks you to plan a meeting to plan his care after discharge. What is this type of meeting called?*

Case 3

While working in a Community Mental Health Team, you are asked to visit a 22-year-old man, Tom, at home. His concerned mother has contacted services. She reports that he dropped out of college two years ago and has become increasingly withdrawn since. He spends most of his day in his bedroom with the curtains drawn, muttering to himself about cars which stop outside the house. He is reluctant to talk to you, but eventually confides that he believes red cars follow him whenever he goes out, monitoring his movements because they want to kill him. He recently saw a red car parked at a bus stop and believed this was a message from MI5 telling him to 'watch out'. He has smoked cannabis regularly since the age of 14, but less so in the last year. The longest he has abstained from cannabis use was three months, but this made little difference to his symptoms. His mother tells you worry about her son is driving the family apart.

1 *What psychotic symptoms are described?*
2 *What is the most likely diagnosis?*

You discuss the patient at the next CMHT meeting and a care coordinator is allocated. She wishes to discuss a care plan for him.

3 *What do you think are the priorities for his treatment?*

Tom reluctantly agrees to take antipsychotics. He has no relevant medical history. You decide to prescribe olanzapine.

4 *List three important side-effects of this drug.*
5 *Tom's mother is concerned to know whether he will get better. What can you tell her about the prognosis?*
6 *Tom's mother asks what she and Tom can do to maximize the chances of him getting and staying well.*

Case 4

A 16-year-old girl attends a GP surgery with her mother, who is concerned about her daughter's significant weight loss. She looks thin and pale.

1 *Name four common conditions, at least two of which are psychiatric, that may have caused this weight loss.*

On physical examination, she is found to be very thin. She is 159 cm tall and weighs 40 kg. Her pulse is 56. There are no abnormal clinical signs. She has a Hb of 10.2, albumin of 30 and potassium of 3.0. Otherwise, blood investigations are unremarkable.

2 *What is her body mass index (BMI)? What does this indicate?*
3 *What other questions might the GP ask at this stage?*

The answers of the patient and her mother lead you to conclude she has anorexia nervosa.

4 *How would you manage her condition?*
5 *What factors would you consider in deciding whether she should be treated as an inpatient or an outpatient?*

Treatment is unsuccessful and her weight falls to 33 kg over the next six months. Her potassium level also falls to 1.9 and you are seriously concerned for her life. She is refusing all food. She tells you she is indifferent as to whether she lives or dies, her main concern is to be thin. She refuses to let you insert a nasogastric tube to feed her.

6 *Can you insert the nasogastric tube? If so, under what legal authority?*

Case 5

Monica is 19 years old and has recently arrived in the UK from Uganda. She is claiming political asylum. She has been brought to the A&E department by a fellow resident at the hostel where she is staying because she has become increasingly agitated and fearful. She tells you that 'the rebels are after me' and her agitation increases markedly each time there is a loud noise.

1 *What possible diagnoses are you considering at this point?*

Monica tells you that six months ago her family home was broken into by rebel soldiers who killed her parents in front of her and then forced her to go with them to a military camp. She was made to be the 'concubine' of one of the rebel leaders who raped her repeatedly. She finally escaped with the help of one of the rebel soldiers.

2 *Does this history support the diagnosis of PTSD? What other questions would you ask to help confirm the diagnosis?*

Monica says that she often thinks about killing herself, but thinks it would be wrong and that it would upset the friends who have supported her since she came to the UK.

3 *What other questions would you ask to assess her risk of suicide?*
4 *How would you manage Monica's PTSD?*

Case 6

Jim is 80 years old and has had no recent health problems. He attends the GP surgery with his wife. According to Jim there is nothing the matter, but his wife says that for the past year he has become increasingly forgetful. Though he is normally an excellent driver, the previous day Jim had ignored a no entry sign while driving back from their daughter's house and only narrowly avoided crashing the car.

1 *What diagnostic possibilities would you consider?*

2 *What questions would you ask Jim and his wife before proceeding to a physical examination?*

Jim repeats that he has no problems at all. His wife tells you that over the past year she has taken over most of the tasks that had been his responsibility throughout their marriage, such as paying bills and arranging for the car to be serviced. He can no longer use the TV remote control properly. He has never been physically aggressive, but he sometimes shouts at his wife when he is at his most confused and frustrated. She finds it difficult to cope with his changing personality, his lack of initiative and his loss of active interest in her and their family.

3 *What features would you look for particularly in the examination of the mental state and the physical examination?*
4 *What tests would you order and why?*

Jim's MMSE score is 18/30, indicating moderate cognitive impairment. He performs particularly badly on short-term memory. He is only able to name six animals in a minute and only four fruits. His pulse is 60 and regular, his blood pressure is 120/75, fundoscopy is normal and there are no abnormal neurological signs. He has a small smooth goitre.

The CT scan shows generalized atrophy. All other results are normal.

5 *What is the likeliest diagnosis?*

Case 7

As a psychiatric junior doctor, you see Andrew, a 12-year-old boy who has been brought to clinic by his parents. They have become increasingly concerned about his behaviour, which has deteriorated over the last year since he moved to senior school. They asked his GP for help after Andrew was warned by the police for attempting to set fire to an abandoned car on the local recreation ground with his friends. At a recent parents' evening, his form teacher also expressed concern that he seemed to be having difficulty concentrating, and is over-talkative in class, which distracts the other students. She commented that he seems to have developed a tic, which involves Andrew blinking his eyes, which his mother says dates back a few years. He is bullied at school.

His parents adopted Andrew when he was five years old, and have been told that his birth mother had alcohol and opiate dependence and mental health problems. There is no information on the biological father. As a young child Andrew was overactive and clumsy. When you see Andrew, he avoids making eye contact and is very reluctant to engage. He admits to feeling annoyed and sad. He says he hates life.

1 *Give at least four possible diagnoses.*

After a full investigation, you diagnose him with ADHD.

2 *How could you treat this?*

You see Andrew in clinic with his mother a few months later. His ADHD is slightly improved with treatment, but he feels very sad and is sleeping poorly. You diagnose him with depression.

3 *How would you treat this?*
4 *His mother remains concerned about the tic he has developed. What further information would help you clarify the diagnosis.*

Case 8

A 25-year-old woman lives with her mother and half-sister who has bipolar affective disorder. She was referred by her GP after she told him at a routine appointment that she often has an overwhelming impulse to jump in front of a train when she is standing at a station. This has alarmed her as she does not want to die. She has never harmed herself and has never wanted to. She has recently lost her job due to consistent poor time-keeping. Although she wakes several hours before she needs to leave the house, she cannot bear to leave until she has washed herself at least five times. If she touches the floor with her bare feet after her shower she has to start again. If she does not do this the thoughts of being contaminated with dirt become unbearable. She comments that she knows her thoughts are 'not logical' and feels frustrated that she cannot stop her excessive washing.

1 *What is the risk of suicide in this patient?*
2 *What is the most likely diagnosis?*

You want to find out if the patient has other symptoms of OCD that she has not mentioned yet.

3 *What other potential symptoms might you ask about?*
4 *What is the initial management of OCD?*
5 *You tell the patient you would like to refer her for CBT. She asks you what the therapy might involve. What would you tell her?*
6 *What is the prognosis of OCD?*

Case 9

You are asked to see Mr Tomkins, a 50-year-old living in a hostel for people with chronic mental health problems. The staff there have observed him making strange movements of his mouth and tongue. He denies feeling bothered by these movements, and says that he wants to talk no more about anything. The support worker tells you that he spends most of his day smoking and engages very little with staff or other patients. He needs encouragement to wash. He does not pose any management problems and the staff feel he is quite happy in himself.

Mr Tomkins has lived in the hostel for 20 years. He was placed there after closure of the local psychiatric asylum where he was an inpatient for most of the 1970s. You obtain the old notes and find that he was diagnosed with paranoid schizophrenia in 1975. He has not had any delusions or hallucinations for over five years. His current medication is procyclidine 5 mg tds and haloperidol decanoate (depot) im 150 mg every four weeks. This has been decreased gradually from a dose of 300 mg every four weeks during his last admission five years ago.

1 *What is the most likely psychiatric diagnosis and why?*
2 *Why do you think the patient was prescribed procyclidine?*
3 *The Support worker has noticed the strange movements develop over the last six months and asks what is causing them. What do you tell him?*
4 *How could you treat his movement disorder?*
5 *Give two advantages and two disadvantages of depot medication compared with taking tablets.*

Case 10

Mary is 61 years old. She initially presented to the GP surgery three months ago with a six-month history of increasingly low mood, poor appetite and loss of energy. A diagnosis of depression was made and she was started on citalopram 20 mg. She says that she is feeling no better.

1 *What are the key questions you would ask her before formulating a management plan?*

Mary tells you that she has taken the citalopram every day. She has fleeting thoughts that she would be better off dead, but that she would never act on them because it would hurt her children too much. She worries constantly about them, and also about her elderly father who is in a care home and for the past year has no longer been able to recognize her when she visits. She adds that her husband was initially very supportive, but has now become impatient with her, partly (she thinks) because she has no interest whatever in sex. She has had no particular physical symptoms apart from those described. Despite her poor appetite she has gained 2 kg in the past three months.

2 *Is there any need to do a physical examination or take blood tests?*

There are no significant abnormalities on physical examination and Mary's thyroid function tests are normal.

3 *What options might you consider for managing Mary's continuing depression?*

OSCE examiner mark sheets

Station 1

☐ Polite and appropriate introduction

☐ Demonstrates empathy

☐ Use of appropriate language (avoiding excessive technical language and explaining terms used)

☐ Ascertained existing level of knowledge

☐ Asked patient for feedback about whether information understandable/answered the question

☐ Responds to verbal and non-verbal cues

☐ Offers leaflets or further source of information

1. What does bipolar affective disorder mean?

☐ Episodic illness, well between episodes

☐ Mood disorder

☐ Depressive episodes

☐ Manic episodes (increased mood, feelings of increased abilities or esteem, decreased sleep, reckless or impulsive behaviour)

2. Why are blood tests needed when taking lithium?

☐ Renal function

☐ Thyroid function

☐ Monitor level of lithium

☐ Brief, reasonable explanation for blood tests – ensure safe but adequate levels OR to detect renal/thyroid problems so can be managed

3. What should the patient do if she wants to stop taking the medication? Will she be sectioned if she stops without discussing it first?

☐ Advise to consult GP if she has concerns about medication

☐ Consider other medication OR reducing gradually

☐ Would not section someone who was well because they had stopped taking medication

☐ More likely to have a further episode if stop medication

☐ If mental health, safety or safety of others serious concern and refusing treatment, would be assessed under Mental Health Act

4. What should the patient do about medication if she wants to get pregnant?

☐ Talk to doctor as early as possible, preferably before trying to conceive

☐ Potential risk to unborn child from lithium

☐ Need to balance risks from medication against need to stay well

Station 2

☐ Polite and appropriate introduction

☐ Demonstrates empathy

☐ Appropriate use of silence to give time to talk

☐ Responding to verbal and non-verbal cues

☐ Good balance of open and closed questions

☐ Current suicidal ideation

☐ Whether method of self-harm considered

☐ Elicited availability of method

☐ Assessed current suicidal intent

☐ Asked about protective factors

☐ Asked whether would feel able to talk to someone if intent returned

☐ Assessed risk of harm to child

☐ Assessed risk of child neglect/elicited that husband/mother helping

How do you think this risk should be managed?

☐ Crisis team

☐ Ongoing monitoring

Do you think it is safe for Charlie to stay at home while she is unwell?

☐ Yes

 Psychiatry at a Glance, 4e. By C. Katona, C. Cooper and M. Robertson. Published 2008 Blackwell Publishing. ISBN: 978-1-4501-8117-4

Answers to EMQs

1. Treatment in psychiatry
1d
2c
3h
4g
5e

2. Epidemiology in psychiatry
1a
2g
3c
4e
5b
6a
7b

3. Psychiatry and the law
1c
2j
3k
4a
5e
6f
7i

4. Substance misuse
1g
2d
3k
4f
5a
6c
7e

5. Mental state
1a
2i
3c
4j
5f
6h
7g

6. Delusions
1a
2j
3c
4e
5g
6h
7b

7. Psychiatric treatment
1h
2c
3d
4k
5f
6a
7e
8i

8. Cognitive impairment
1g
2d
3b
4f
5h
6e
7c

9. Personality disorders
1g
2c
3e
4i
5d
6e
7b

10. Child and adolescent psychiatry
1i
2d
3g
4a
5b
6c
7j

Psychiatry at a Glance, 4e. By C. Katona, C. Cooper and M. Robertson. Published 2008 Blackwell Publishing. ISBN: 978-1-4501-8117-4 **103**

Answers to case studies

Case 1

1 Persecutory delusions; visual hallucinations
2 Acute confusional state; the history of an acute onset, and the fluctuating level of confusion are typical of an acute confusional state; other symptoms suggestive of this are irritability, incoherent speech, visual hallucinations (police officer) and persecutory delusions.
3 The history is suggestive of chronic pulmonary disease, so a chest infection is a likely cause in this case; urinary tract infection is also a very common cause of confusion. Other common causes include alcohol withdrawal, hypoxia, electrolyte disturbance (e.g. hyponatraemia) (see Chapter 31 for more).
4 Non-pharmacological measures would include reassurance, nursing in a well-lit room, avoiding frequent changes of staff, ensuring glasses and hearing aid were available if she uses them.
5 Avoid drug treatment if possible, but if required to prevent severe distress or risk of harm to others, a benzodiazepine (e.g. lorazepam) would be a first choice.
6 She should be assessed for a section 5(2), and detained if thought to be at risk of harm to herself or others if she left the ward. A Mental Health Act assessment could then be arranged.

Case 2

1 Although three months after the death of his partner normal grieving would be expected, because of his negative thoughts about himself and his life and severe suicidal risk this would appear to meet criteria for a (severe) depressive episode.
2 High; he has recently made a serious attempt on his life, nothing has changed since then and he says he wants to die. He is depressed, unemployed, male, socially isolated and has been diagnosed with HIV – all of these are risk factors for suicide.
3 Recently bereaved people without mental illness often report visual pseudo-hallucinations and hallucinations of the dead person and these should not be pathologized (see Chapter 10). However, as he has a severe depression, you should be alert for other symptoms which may indicate the development of a psychotic depression.
4 Antidepressants. Psychological treatment (e.g. cognitive behavioural therapy) of his depression would also be indicated. Membership of a support organization for people with HIV could also be helpful.
5 He would most likely be placed under section 2, because he has no psychiatric history and the admission would be for assessment of his psychiatric disorder. If he had an established diagnosis of depression, section 3 would be appropriate.
6 A Care Programme Approach (CPA) meeting.

Case 3

1 Persecutory delusions, delusional perception and delusions of reference.
2 Schizophrenia. The psychotic symptoms have been present for over a month, as required by ICD-10 criteria for schizophrenia. Although he has smoked cannabis, his symptoms do not occur in the context of cannabis use alone.
3 Engaging Tom and encouraging him to accept antipsychotic medication. Psychoeducation regarding the likely role of cannabis in exacerbating his symptoms. Returning to social, academic or work commitments is an important component of recovery, and encour-

agement to do this when he is able can be given. Family therapy and CBT may be appropriate.
4 Weight gain, glucose intolerance, sedation.
5 After a first psychotic episode there is a 90% chance of being well within a year, but about an 80% chance of a further episode within five years. His psychosis has been untreated for up to two years which may worsen prognosis (see Chapter 7).
6 The main factors likely to influence the outcome will be whether Tom takes his antipsychotic medication consistently, refrains from smoking cannabis and avoids undue stress; there is some suggestion of high levels of stress in the family and family therapy to address this might also improve outcome.

Case 4

1 Psychiatric conditions: anorexia nervosa, depression, substance misuse; physical conditions: diabetes mellitus, acute or chronic infection, malabsorption (e.g. coeliac disease) (list not exhaustive).
2 BMI = $40/1.59^2$ = 15.8. This indicates she is severely underweight. A diagnosis of anorexia nervosa requires a BMI <17.5, in association with other diagnostic factors.
3 Anorexia nervosa by this point is a likely diagnosis, as no other physical cause has been found and blood parameters are consistent with decreased food intake. Key questions would be to determine if the weight loss is deliberate, whether the girl has a morbid fear of fatness, and amenorrhea.
4 Psychological approaches that have demonstrated effectiveness in treating anorexia nervosa include family therapy, cognitive behavioural therapy and interpersonal psychotherapy.
5 Treatment is as an outpatient, unless there are risks to her mental health (from suicide) or physical health (e.g. severe hypokalaemia); at BMI <13.5 the risk of death from fatal arrhythmias or hypoglcaemia is high; inability to rise without support from a squat also indicates severe physical frailty that would require admission.
6 Yes; treatment of anorexia nervosa through refeeding may take place under the provisions of the Mental Health Act (usually section 3) since it is regarded as being treatment of the mental illness.

Case 5

1 The presenting complaint about the rebels raises the possibility of a delusional disorder, but the fact that she is an asylum seeker (and therefore likely to be escaping from persecution) and her hypervigilance suggest the possibility of post-traumatic stress disorder (PTSD).
2 Yes, what Monica has experienced is clearly of an 'exceptionally threatening or catastrophic nature, which is likely to cause pervasive distress in almost anyone'. You should ask Monica whether she experiences dreams or daytime 'flashbacks', and whether she feels 'numb' and less responsive than she used to be to other people or her surroundings. Does she avoid situations that remind her of her past traumatic experiences? Is her sleep poor? Has she ever thought of harming herself?
3

• Previous attempts and associated intent to die.
• Current feelings of hopelessness.
• Specific current plans (method, putting affairs in order).

- Extent to which suicidal thoughts would be influenced by asylum status (threat of removal, granting of leave to remain).
4 SSRI antidepressants, Eye Movement Desensitization and Reprogramming and trauma-focused psychotherapy have all been shown to be effective whereas the effects of anxiolytic drugs and of debriefing are less clear. Resolution of Monica's symptoms will be difficult while her asylum status remains uncertain.

Case 6

1 The forgetfulness with gradual onset and the apparently reduced competence in a complex task (driving) suggest a dementia syndrome. The commonest causes of dementia are Alzheimer's disease and vascular dementia, but dementia with Lewy bodies and alcohol-related dementia are also relatively common. The apparent sudden worsening in cognitive function also suggests the possibility of an acute confusional state (delirium). This could be secondary to a stroke, a myocardial infarction or an acute (respiratory or urinary) infection
2 Your questions should attempt to establish whether Jim has lost competence in other daily living skills, to narrow down the diagnostic possibilities and also to assess risk. What are the main problems from his wife's point of view? Does he have any problems with washing, dressing, managing money, etc.? Has he had any previous episodes of sudden confusion or of unilateral loss of power or coordination? Has he ever put himself or his wife at risk by his behaviour (e.g. getting lost, leaving pans to boil dry)? Has he ever been verbally or physically aggressive towards his wife (see Chapter 4)? Does he ever seem suspicious or express delusional ideas? Is there any suggestion of auditory or visual hallucinations?
3 Systematic assessment of cognitive function is essential and using a standardized screen such as the Mini Mental State Examination can be helpful. The change in personality suggests the possibility of frontal lobe involvement so frontal lobe tests such as verbal fluency may be revealing (see Chapter 2). On physical examination it is important to examine blood pressure and look for evidence of vascular disease (weak or absent pulses, fundal examination), of lateralizing neurological signs, Parkinsonian features and signs of hypothyroidism.
4 The most informative test is a CT or MRI scan which may show generalized atrophy suggestive of Alzheimer's disease, and/or cortical or subcortical infarction. Other useful tests include TFTs (because of the bradycardia and goitre), ECG (to exclude recent myocardial infarction), full blood count (anaemia may aggravate cognitive impairment) and urea and electrolytes (both because he is on a diuretic and because renal failure can worsen cognitive function) (see Chapter 31 for full confusion screen).
5 Alzheimer's disease.

Case 7

1 Attention deficit hyperactivity disorder; conduct disorder; Tourette's syndrome; depression.
2 Stimulants (e.g. methylphenidate); atomoxetine; behavioural therapy; parent training in behavioural methods (e.g. Webster–Stratton parenting programme).
3 Psychological therapies (e.g. CBT) are the main treatment. Antidepressants are not generally recommended for children under 18, although they are prescribed for severe or resistant cases by specialists.
4 If the motor tic described has been present, together with one or more vocal tics, for at least a year, this would fulfil the diagnostic criteria for Tourette's disorder.

Case 8

1 Low; there are no suicidal thoughts, intent or plans and no history of self-harm. The thought of jumping in front of a train is an obsessional impulse rather than a suicidal thought because she experiences it as unwelcome and she tries to resist it.
2 Obsessive compulsive disorder (OCD) – she gives a clear history of obsessional thoughts, impulses and compulsions that occupy several hours each day. Her thoughts are ego-dystonic (i.e. they are unwelcome and she tries to resist them). This is important in differentiating OCD from a psychotic disorder.
3 Obsessional images or other obsessional thoughts (e.g. regarding sex, blasphemy); other compulsions such as checking (e.g. the gas), counting, touching and constant rearrangement of objects to achieve symmetry; hoarding or excessive tidiness (see Chapter 12).
4 OCD can respond well to SSRIs or clomipramine, together with cognitive behaviour therapy.
5 The therapist will discuss her symptoms in detail and with her to identify those that are causing her most distress. In her case this may well be the excessive hand-washing. The therapist will then design a programme with her of graded exposure and response prevention (see Chapter 33).
6 Chronic, with waxing and waning of symptoms. Patients with compulsions only, those with severe symptoms, persistent life stresses or premorbid obsessionality fare worst.

Case 9

1 Residual or chronic schizophrenia. He had paranoid schizophrenia years ago, with delusions and hallucinations, but for the last five years he has not had these 'positive symptoms' (see Chapter 6). He exhibits a number of negative symptoms of schizophrenia: lack of motivation, social withdrawal and lack of concern for social conventions.
2 Procyclidine is prescribed to treat the Parkinsonian side-effects often caused by typical antipsychotics (see Chapter 34).
3 That the movements are known as tardive dyskinesia and are often seen in people who have been on long-term treatment with typical antipsychotics; long-term use of haloperidol is the most likely cause in this case.
4 His depot medication could be gradually reduced further, and the procyclidine could also be reduced. Tetrabenazine is sometimes helpful if these measures do not improve the symptoms.
5 Advantages: the patient does not need to remember to take tablets; adherence to treatment can be monitored more reliably. Disadvantages: having injections can be unpleasant; there may be problems with the injection site as for all injections; many patients find the experience disempowering.

Case 10

1 You need to assess how severe her depression is and whether there is a significant risk of suicide. You should ask whether her mood still changes with external circumstances, whether she has feelings of hopelessness and whether she has any suicidal thoughts or plans. You need to know whether she takes the citalopram as prescribed and if not, what her reasons are. These might include fear of addiction and side-effects. It is also important to enquire about any physical or psychological factors that may be preventing her recovery (e.g. recent bereavement or other life stresses or poorly controlled pain). Does she have any physical symptoms suggestive of underlying malignancy?

2 Mary's loss of energy and weight gain raise the possibility of hypo-thyroidism, which is particularly common in post-menopausal women. Hypothyroidism can make depression more resistant to treatment so it is important to check her pulse, examine her neck and order thyroid function tests.

3 You have identified potentially important psychological 'mainte-nance factors' – Mary's worries about her father and her husband's impatience. Mary might benefit from attending a carers' group to share her experiences as a carer with others in the same position. It might be helpful (with Mary's permission) to talk to her husband (or preferably to the two of them together) about her depression and in particular about the problems that have arisen in their relationship. More fundamental relationship problems might also be revealed. A number of pharmacological approaches should also be considered. These include increasing the dose of citalopram, changing to another class of antidepressant (such as an SNRI or mirtazapine) or adding a second drug such as lithium carbonate.

Further reading

Chapters 1–3

APA (2002) *Diagnostic and Statistical Manual of Mental Disorder*, 4th edn text revision. American Psychiatric Association, Washington, DC.

Kendell, R. E. (2001) The distinction between mental and physical illness. *British Journal of Psychiatry*, 178, 490–493.

Maj, M. (2005) 'Psychiatric comorbidity': an artefact of current diagnostic systems? *British Journal of Psychiatry*, 186, 182–184.

Sims, A. (2002) *Symptoms in the Mind*, 3rd edn. Elsevier, Amsterdam.

WHO (2002) *The ICD-10 Classification of Mental and Behavioural Disorders*. World Health Organization, Geneva (www.who.int/classifications/apps/icd/icd10online/).

Chapter 4

Friedman, R. A. (2006) Violence and mental illness – How strong is the link? *New England Journal of Medicine*, 355, 2064–2066.

Morgan, J. (2007) 'Giving up the culture of blame': risk assessment and risk management in psychiatric practice. Briefing document for Royal College of Psychiatrists, London. www.rcpsych.ac.uk/PDF/Risk%20Assessment%20Paper%20-%20Giving%20up%20the%20Culture%20of%20Blame.pdf

Chapter 5

Broadhurst, M. and Gill, P. (2007) Repeated self-injury from a liaison psychiatry perspective. *Advances in Psychiatric Treatment*, 13, 228–235.

Fagin, L. (2006) Repeated self-injury: perspectives from general psychiatry. *Advances in Psychiatric Treatment*, 12, 193–201.

Jordan, J. R. and McMenamy, J. (2004) Interventions for suicide survivors: a review of the literature. *Suicide and Life-Threatening Behaviour*, 4, 337–349.

The National Confidential Inquiry (NCI) into Suicide and Homicide by People with Mental Illness (2006). http://www.medicine.manchester.ac.uk/suicideprevention/nci/

NICE Guidelines on self-harm (2004) http://www.nice.org.uk/pdf/CG016NICEguideline.pdf

Chapters 6 and 7

Davies, E. J. (2007) Developmental aspects of schizophrenia and related disorders: possible implications for treatment strategies. *Advances in Psychiatric Treatment*, 13, 384–391.

Cecile (2005) The environment and schizophrenia: the role of cannabis use. *Schizophr Bull.* July 31(3), 608–612.

McGlashan, T. H. (2005) Early detection and intervention in psychosis: an ethical paradigm shift. *British Journal of Psychiatry*, 187, s113–s115.

McGrath, J., Saha, S., Welham, J. et al. (2004) A systematic review of the incidence of schizophrenia: the distribution of rates and the influence of sex, urbanicity, migrant status and methodology. *BMC Medicine*, 28(2), 13.

Mueser, K. T. and McGurk, S. R. (2004) Schizophrenia. *Lancet*, 19(363) (9426), 2063–2072.

NICE guidelines on schizophrenia (2002) http://www.nice.org.uk/pdf/CG1NICEguideline.pdf

Chapter 8

Ferrier, I. N. (2001) Characterizing the ideal antidepressant therapy to achieve remission. *Journal of Clinical Psychiatry*, 62 (Suppl. 26), 10–15.

Katona, C., Peveler, R., Dowrick, C. et al. (2005) Pain symptoms in depression: definition and clinical significance. *Clin Med.* July–August 5(4), 390–395.

Langlands, R. L., Jorm, A. F., Kelly, C. M. and Kitchener, B. A. (2008) First aid for depression: a Delphi consensus study with consumers, carers and clinicians. *Journal of Affective Disorders*, 105, 157–165.

NICE guidelines on depression (2004) http://www.nice.org.uk/pdf/CG023quickrefguide.pdf

Wolpert, L. (1998) *Malignant Sadness*. Faber, London.

Chapter 9

Angst, J. (2007) The bipolar spectrum. *British Journal of Psychiatry*, 190: 189–191.

Benazzi, F. (2007) Bipolar II disorder: epidemiology, diagnosis and management. *CNS Drugs*, 21(9), 727–740.

Mitchell, P. B. and Malhi, G. S. (2004) Bipolar depression: phenomenological overview and clinical characteristics. *Bipolar Disorders*, 6, 530–539.

Chapter 10

Adshead, G. and Ferris, S. (2007) Treatment of victims of trauma. *Advances in Psychiatric Treatment*, 13, 358–368.

Bisson, J. I. (2007) Post-traumatic stress disorder. *BMJ*, 334, 789–793.

Frueh, B. C., Buckley, T. C., Cusack, K. J. et al. (2004) Cognitive–behavioral treatment for PTSD among people with severe mental illness: a proposed treatment model. *Journal of Psychiatric Practice*, 10(1), 26–38.

NICE guidelines on post-traumatic stress disorder (2006) http://guidance.nice.org.uk/CG26/guidance/pdf/English

Vanderwerker, L. C., Jacobs, S. C., Parkes, C. M. and Prigerson, H. G. (2006) An exploration of associations between separation anxiety in childhood and complicated grief in later life. *J Nerv Ment Dis.*, February, 194(2), 121–123.

Chapter 11

Fricchione, G. (2004) Generalised anxiety disorder. *New England Journal of Medicine*, 351, 675–682.

Katon, W. J. (2006) Panic disorder. *New England Journal of Medicine*, 354, 2360–2367.

Schneier, F. R. (2006) Social anxiety disorder. *New England Journal of Medicine*, 355, 1029–1036.

Chapter 12

Leckman, J. F., Rauch, S. L. and Mataix-Cols, D. (2007) Symptom dimensions in obsessive-compulsive disorder: implications for the DSM-V. *CNS Spectr.*, May, 12(5), 376–387, 400.

NICE guidelines: Obsessive compulsive disorder (2006) http://guidance.nice.org.uk/CG31/guidance/pdf/English

Stein, D. J. (2002) Obsessive-compulsive disorder. *Lancet*, 360(9330), 397–405.

Chapter 13

Gowers, S. G. and Shore, A. (2001) Development of weight and shape concerns in the aetiology of eating disorders. *British Journal of Psychiatry*, 179, 236–242.

Hudson, J. I., Hiripi, E., Pope, H. G. and Kessler, R. C. (2007) The prevalence and correlates of eating disorders in the National Comorbidity Survey replication. *Biological Psychiatry*, 1, 61(3), 348–358.

Jacobi, C., Hayward, C., de Zwaan, M. et al. (2004) Coming to terms with risk factors for eating disorders: Application of risk terminology and suggestions for a general taxonomy. *Psychological Bulletin*, 130, 19–65.

NICE guidelines on eating disorders (2004) http://www.nice.org.uk/pdf/cg009niceguidance.pdf

Treasure, J. and Schmidt, U. (2005) Anorexia nervosa. *Clin Evid.* December (14), 1140–1148. Review.

Chapter 14

Fonagy, P. and Bateman, A. (2006) Progress in the treatment of borderline personality disorder. *British Journal of Psychiatry*, 188, 1–3.

Howells, K., Krishnan, G. and Daffern, M. (2007) Challenges in the treatment of dangerous and severe personality disorder. *Advances in Psychiatric Treatment*, 13, 325–332.

Paris, J. (2004) Borderline or bipolar? Distinguishing borderline personality disorder from bipolar spectrum disorders. *Harvard Review of Psychiatry*, 12(3), 140–145.

Tyrer, P., Coombs, N., Ibrahimi, F. et al. (2007) Critical developments in the assessment of personality disorder. *Br J Psychiatry*, May, 49 (Suppl.), s51–s59.

Chapter 15

Leiblum, S. R. (1998) Definition and classification of female sexual disorders. *International Journal of Impotence Research*, 10 (Suppl. 2), S104–S106.

Lindau, S. T., Schumm, L. P., Laumann, E. O. et al. (2007) A study of sexuality and health among older adults in the United States. *New England Journal of Medicine*, 357, 762–774.

Meston, C. M. and Bradford, A. (2007) Sexual dysfunctions in women. *Annu Rev Clin Psychol*, 3, 233–256.

Wylie, K. (2004) Gender-related disorders. *BMJ (Clinical Research Ed.)*, 11 (329), 615–617.

Chapter 16

Asher, R. (1951) Munchausen's syndrome. *Lancet*, i, 339–341.

Enoch, M. D. and Trethowan, W. (1991) *Uncommon Psychiatric Syndromes*. Butterworth Heinemann, Oxford.

Lepping, P., Russell, P. and Freudenmann, R. W. (2007) Antipsychotic treatment of primary delusional parasitosis: systematic review. *British Journal of Psychiatry*, 191, 198–205.

Chapters 17 and 18

Ball, D. (2004) Genetic approaches to alcohol dependence. *British Journal of Psychiatry*, 185, 449–451.

Department of Health (2007) *Drug Misuse and Dependence – Guidelines on Clinical Management*. HMSO, London. http://www.dh.gov.uk/en/Policyandguidance/Healthandsocialcaretopics/Substancemisuse/Substancemisusegeneralinformation/DH_4064342

Luty, J. (2006) What works in alcohol use disorders? *Advances in Psychiatric Treatment*, 12, 13–22.

Seivewright, N., McMahon, C. and Egleston, P. (2005) Stimulant use still going strong: revisited . . . misuse of amphetamines and related drugs. *Advances in Psychiatric Treatment*, 11(4), 262–269.

Tupala, E. and Tiihonen, J. (2004) Dopamine and alcoholism: neurobiological basis of ethanol abuse. *Progress in Neuro-psychopharmacology and Biological Psychiatry*, 28(8), 1221–1247.

Chapters 19–21

Bushra, H. (2007) Anti-social adolescents conduct disorder: a review. *Community Pract*, July 80(7), 38–40.

Friedman, R. A. (2006) Uncovering an epidemic – screening for mental illness in teens. *New England Journal of Medicine*, 355, 2717–2719.

Maughan, B. and Kim-Cohen, J. (2005) Continuities between childhood and adult life. *British Journal of Psychiatry*, 187, 301–303.

McClure, I. and Le Couteur, A. (2007) Evidence-based approaches to autism spectrum disorders. *Child Care Health Dev*, 33, 509–512.

NICE (2005) guidelines on depression in children and young people. http://guidance.nice.org.uk/CG28/niceguidance/pdf/English

Robertson M. M. (2006) Attention deficit hyperactivity disorder, tics and Tourette's syndrome: the relationship and treatment implications. A commentary. *European Child and Adolescent Psychiatry*, 15, 1–11.

Taylor, E., Dopfner, M., Sergeant J. et al. (2004) European clinical guidelines for hyperkinetic disorder – first upgrade. *Eur Child Adolesc Psychiatry*, 13 (Suppl), 17–30.

Thapar, A., Langley, K., Asherson, P. and Gill, M. (2007) Gene–environment interplay in attention-deficit hyperactivity disorder and the importance of a developmental perspective. *British Journal of Psychiatry*, 190, 1–3.

Chapter 22

Hassiotis, A. and Hall, I. (2004) Behavioural and cognitive–behavioural interventions for outwardly-directed aggressive behaviour in people with learning disabilities. *Cochrane Database of Systematic Reviews (Online)*, 18(4), CD003406.

Kwok, H. and Cheung, P. W. (2007) Co-morbidity of psychiatric disorder and medical illness in people with intellectual disabilities. *Current Opinion in Psychiatry*, 20, 443–449.

Chapter 23

Bhui, K., Stansfeld, S., Hull, S. et al. (2003) Ethnic variations in pathways to and use of specialist mental health services in the UK. Systematic review. *Br J Psychiatry*, February, 182, 105–116.

Bhugra, D. and Mastrogianni, A. (2004) Globalisation and mental disorders: overview with relation to depression. *British Journal of Psychiatry*, 184, 10–20.

Littlewood, R. and Lipsedge, M. (1997) *Aliens and Alienists: Ethnic Minorities and Psychiatry*, 3rd edn. Routledge, London.

Morgan, C. and Fearon, P. (2007) Social experience and psychosis insights from studies of migrant and ethnic minority groups. *Epidemiol Psichiatr Soc*. April–June 16(2), 118–123.

Sumathipala, A., Siribaddana, S. H. and Bhugra, D. (2004) Culture-bound syndromes: the story of dhat syndrome. *British Journal of Psychiatry*, 184, 200–210.

Chapter 24

Birmingham, L. (2003) The mental health of prisoners. *Advances in Psychiatric Treatment*, 9, 191–199.

Fazel, M., Wheeler, J. and Danesh, J. (2005) Prevalence of serious mental disorder in 7000 refugees resettled in western countries: a systematic review. *Lancet*, 365(9467), 1309–1314.

Grenier, P. (1996) *Still Dying for a Home*. Crisis, London.

Killaspy, H., Ritchie, C., Greer, E. and Robertson, M. (2004) Treating the homeless mentally ill: does a designated inpatient facility improve outcome? *Journal of Mental Health*, 13, 593–599.

Royal College of Psychiatrists (2006) Improving services for refugees and asylum seekers: position statement. www.rcpsych.ac.uk/docs/R efugee%20asylum%20seeker%20consensus%20final.doc

Tribe, R. (2002) Mental health of refugees and asylum-seekers. *Advances in Psychiatric Treatment*, 8, 242–249.

Chapter 25

Boath, E., Bradley, E. and Henshaw, C. (2005) The prevention of postnatal depression: a narrative systematic review. *J Psychosom Obstet Gynaecol*. September, 26(3), 185–192.

Day, E. and George, S. (2005) Management of drug misuse in pregnancy. *Advances in Psychiatric Treatment*, 11, 253–261.

Kohen, D. (2004) Psychotropic medication in pregnancy. *Advances in Psychiatric Treatment*, 10, 59–66.

Oates, M. (2003) Suicide: the leading cause of maternal death. *British Journal of Psychiatry*, 183, 279–282.

Chapter 26

Alexopoulos, G. S. (2006) The vascular depression hypothesis: 10 years later. *Biol Psychiatry*. December, 60(12), 1304–1305.

Baldwin, R., Graham, G., Chiu, E. and Katona, C. (2002) *Guidelines on Depression in Older People – Practising the Evidence*. Martin Dunitz, London.

Karim, S. and Byrne, E. J. (2005) Treatment of psychosis in elderly people. *Advances in Psychiatric Treatment*, 11, 286–296.

Katona, C. and Livingston, G. (2002) How well do antidepressants work in older people? A systematic review of number needed to treat. *Journal of Affective Disorders*, 69(1–3), 47–52.

Chapter 27

Arolt, V. and Rothermundt, M. (2004) Depression in medical patients. *Advances in Psychosomatic Medicine*, 26, 98–117.

Guthrie, E. (2006) Psychological treatments in liaison psychiatry: the evidence base. *Clinical Medicine*, 6, 544–547.

Owens, C. and Dein, S. (2006) Conversion disorder: the modern hysteria. *Advances in Psychiatric Treatment*, 12, 152–157.

Spence, S. A. (2006) All in the mind? The neural correlates of unexplained physical symptoms. *Advances in Psychiatric Treatment*, 12, 349–358.

Chapters 28–30

Butler, R. (2006) Prion diseases in humans: an update. *British Journal of Psychiatry*, 189, 295–296.

Dilley, M. and Fleminger, S. (2006) Advances in neuropsychiatry: clinical implications. *Advances in Psychiatric Treatment*, 12, 23–34.

Freeman, M., Patel, V., Collins, P. Y. and Bertolote, J. (2005) Integrating mental health in global initiatives for HIV/AIDS. *British Journal of Psychiatry*, 187, 1–3.

Robertson, M. M. (2008) The international prevalence, epidemiology and clinical phenomenology of Gilles de la Tourette syndrome: Part 1 – the epidemiological and prevalence studies. *Journal of Psychosomatic Research*.

Robertson, M. M. (2008) The international prevalence, epidemiology and clinical phenomenology of Gilles de la Tourette syndrome: Part 2 – tentative explanations for differing prevalence figures in GTS including the possible effects of psychopathology, aetiology, cultural differences and differing phenotypes. *Journal of Psychosomatic Research*.

Rosenblatt, A. (2007) Neuropsychiatry of Huntington's disease. *Dialogues Clin Neurosci*, 9(2), 191–197.

Scahill, L., Erenberg, G., Berlin, C. M. et al. (2006) Contemporary assessment and pharmacotherapy of Tourette syndrome. *J Am Soc Experimental NeuroTherapeutics*, 3, 192–206.

Chapter 31

Inouye, S. K (2006) Delirium in older persons. *New England Journal of Medicine*, 354, 1157–1165.

Lyketsos, C. G., Kozauer, N. and Rabins, P. V. (2007) Psychiatric manifestations of neurologic disease: where are we headed? *Dialogues Clin Neurosci*, 9(2), 111–124.

Chapter 32

Bayley, J. (1998) *Iris*. Abacus, London.

Blennow, K., de Leon, M. J. and Zetterberg, H. (2006) Alzheimer's disease. *Lancet*. July, 368(9533), 387–403.

Burke, D., Hickie, I., Breakspear, M. and Götz, J. (2007). Possibilities for the prevention and treatment of cognitive impairment and dementia. *British Journal of Psychiatry*, 190, 371–372.

Katona, C., Livingston, G., Cooper, C. et al. (2007) International Psychogeriatric Association consensus statement on defining and measuring treatment benefits in dementia. *Int Psychogeriatr*, June, 19(3), 345–354.

Livingston, G., Cooper, C., Woods, C. et al. (2007) Successful ageing in adversity. The LASER-AD longitudinal study. *J Neurol Neurosurg Psychiatry*, September.

Snowden, J. S., Neary, D. and Mann, D. M. A. (2002) Frontotemporal dementia. *British Journal of Psychiatry*, 180, 140–143.

Stewart, R. (2002) Vascular dementia: a diagnosis running out of time. *British Journal of Psychiatry*, 180, 152–156.

Chapter 33

Robins, C. J. and Chapman, A. L. (2004) Dialectical behavior therapy: current status, recent developments, and future directions. *Journal of Personality Disorders*, 18(1), 73–89.

Rollinson, R., Haig, C. and Warner, R. (2007) The application of cognitive-behavioral therapy for psychosis in clinical and research settings. *Psychiatr Serv*. October, 58(10), 1297–1302.

Chapters 34–37

Christmas, D., Morrison, C. and Eljamel, M. S. (2004) Neurosurgery for mental disorder. *Advances in Psychiatric Treatment*, 10, 189–199.

Cookson, J., Taylor, D. and Katona, C. (2003) *Drugs in Psychiatry*. Gaskell Press, London.

Davis, J. (2006). The choice of drugs for schizophrenia. *New England Journal of Medicine*, 354, 518–520.

Kern, D. and Kumar, R. (2007) Deep brain stimulation. *Neurologist*, 13, 237–252.

Mann, J. J. (2005) The medical management of depression. *New England Journal of Medicine*, 353, 1819–1834.

Scott, A. I. F. (2005). College guidelines on electroconvulsive therapy: an update for prescribers. *Advances in Psychiatric Treatment*, 11, 150–156.

Chapter 38

Cooper, C. and Bebbington, P. (2005) Focus on Mental Health Office of National Statistics. http://www.statistics.gov.uk/downloads/theme_compendia/foh2005/09_MentalHealth.pdf

Lester, H. (2005). Shared care for people with mental illness: a GP's perspective. *Advances in Psychiatric Treatment*, 11, 133–139.

Chapter 39

Coid, J. W. (2002) Personality disorders in prisoners and their motivation for dangerous and disruptive behaviour. *Criminal Behaviour and Mental Health*, 12(3), 209–226.

Haque, Q. and Cumming, I. (2003). Intoxication and legal defences. *Advances in Psychiatric Treatment*, 9, 144–151.

Okai, D., Owen, G., Mcguire, H. et al. (2007) Mental capacity in psychiatric patients: systematic review. *British Journal of Psychiatry*, 191, 291–297.

Shaw, J., Hunt, I. M., Flynn, S. et al. (2006) Rates of mental disorder in people convicted of homicide: national clinical survey. *British Journal of Psychiatry*, 188, 143–147.

Chapters 40–42

Bamford Review of Mental Health and Learning Disability (Northern Ireland) http://www.rmhldni.gov.uk/index/internal-papers.htm

Department of Health (1999) Code of Practice to the Mental Health Act 1983 (revised 1999) www.dh.gov.uk/en/Publicationsandstatistics/Publications/PublicationsPolicyAndGuidance/DH_4005756

Mental Health Act 2007 http://www.opsi.gov.uk/acts/acts2007/pdf/ukpga_20070012_en.pdf

Office of Public Sector Information (2003) Mental Health (Care and Treatment) (Scotland) Act 2003 http://www.opsi.gov.uk/legislation/scotland/acts2003/20030013.htm

Glossary

Affect: the observed external manifestation of emotion (see Chapter 2).

Affective disorder: mood disorder.

Agnosia: a loss of ability to recognize objects, people, sounds, smells or other sensory stimuli which is not due to sensory loss.

Akathisia: an unpleasant subjective feeling of restlessness resulting in an inability to sit still or a need to pace.

Anhedonia: inability to experience enjoyment when taking part in previously enjoyed activities.

Anxiety: subjective experience of worry or fear.

Arithmomania: a compulsion that involves counting (see Chapter 12).

Attention: the ability to focus selectively on a current task.

Automatic negative thoughts: thoughts that influence mood and behaviour that are experienced as coming unbidden into consciousness (e.g. 'They are probably not answering the phone because they hate me'). Cognitive behavioural therapy is based on identifying and challenging such thoughts.

Avoidance: avoiding unpleasant thoughts or actual situations because they cause distress or anxiety.

Behavioural management: a system used to alter undesirable behaviour, usually employed in people with dementia or learning disability. The undesirable behaviour is analysed to determine its Antecedents (A), define the actual Behaviour (B) in detail and explore its Consequences (C). Practical interventions are then implemented to reduce it and their success monitored. For example, to reduce wandering in a person with dementia, an intervention may involve encouraging the carer to increase the amount of exercise the person has during the day, and avoiding napping and caffeine.

Blunted affect: a patient's emotional response is very limited in range; the normal range of emotions (laughing or appearing sad at appropriate times) is not encountered; it is a negative symptom in schizophrenia.

Body dysmorphic disorder: an obsessional belief that parts of one's body are misshapen.

Care coordinator: member of the multidisciplinary team who is responsible for delivery of a patient's care. They review the patient regularly, organize Care Programme Approach meetings and ensure the care plan is carried out.

Care plan: a written treatment plan, usually agreed between health professionals and patients. It may include medication (and monitoring of it), and psychological and social interventions.

Care Programme Approach (CPA): the system by which patients of Community Mental Health Teams are managed through regular (at least six-monthly) meetings at which the patient and health professionals agree a care plan, which is then implemented by a care coordinator.

Catatonia: extreme disorder of motor function which occurs in catatonic schizophrenia; patients may stay still for hours, alternatively there may be periods of extreme motor activity. They may show stereotyped, repetitive movements, bizarre posturing, mutism, echolalia and echopraxia.

Chorea: rapid, jerky, dance-like movement of the body.

Circumstantial speech: speech that is discursive and takes a long time to get to the point.

Community Mental Health Team (CMHT): team of health and social care professionals who together deliver psychiatric services to people living in a defined area.

Compulsions: repetitive, purposeful, physical or mental behaviours performed with reluctance in response to an obsession. They are carried out according to certain rules in a stereotyped fashion, and are designed to neutralize or prevent discomfort or a dreaded event.

Concentration: the ability to maintain attention on a current task. This is often tested in the cognitive examination by asking a patient to spell a word (e.g. 'world') backwards.

Confabulation: a falsified memory; patients with memory loss often confabulate as they cannot remember what has really happened.

Conversion: a synonym for dissociation (see below).

Core belief: central beliefs about oneself and the world that underlie thoughts and behaviours (see Chapter 33).

Counter-transference: the converse of transference, where the therapist experiences strong emotions towards the patient.

Defence mechanisms: psychological strategies employed unconsciously by people to reduce anxiety and feelings of internal conflict. Examples include splitting, denial and projection.

Deliberate self-harm: intentionally self-inflicted harm without a fatal outcome. The action may or may not have been carried out with the intent of causing death.

Delusion: fixed, false, firmly held belief out of keeping with the patient's culture, which is unaltered by evidence to the contrary. Types of delusion include grandiose delusions, persecutory delusions, thought insertion, withdrawal, broadcast, delusions of reference, passivity, somatic passivity, delusional perception and nihilistic delusions.

Delusional perception: a delusion that arises in response to a normal perception (see Chapter 6).

Delusions of grandiosity: a delusional belief that the patient has special abilities, powers or is an important person.

Delusions of guilt: a delusional belief that the patient has committed a terrible crime or other act. May occur in psychotic depression.

Delusions of jealousy/infidelity: a delusional belief that the patient's partner is being unfaithful.

Delusions of nihilism: a delusional belief that the patient has lost all their money, possessions or that they are dead or their body is rotting.

Delusions of persecution: a delusional belief that an organization (e.g. MI5), person or other force is trying to harm the patient.

Delusions of reference: a delusional belief that events have a particular meaning to the patient (e.g. TV programmes are conveying messages, cars parked in the street are there for a special reason pertaining to the patient). The content is comparable to ideas of reference but they are held with delusional intensity.

Depersonalization: the unpleasant experience of subjective change, feeling detached, unreal, empty within, unable to feel emotion, watching oneself from outside (e.g. 'It feels as if I am cut off by a pane of glass').

Derealization: the experience of the world or people in it seeming lifeless ('as if made out of cardboard').

Disinhibition: a loss of social conventions which leads to behaviour that is inappropriate to the social setting (e.g. over-familiarity, type of clothing, sexual behaviour and speech).

Dissociative, dissociation: the process by which psychological distress is experienced as physical (usually in the form of neurological symptoms) (see Chapter 27).

Dual diagnosis: literally, fulfilling criteria for two diagnoses at once; in psychiatry this most often refers to the presence of a substance misuse disorder and a psychiatric disorder concurrently.

Dysmorphophobia: an excessive preoccupation with imagined or barely noticeable defects in physical appearance (e.g. preoccupation with the size of the nose, believing an objectively normal nose to be ugly and deformed).

Dysphasia: difficulty with understanding or verbally communicating. In cognitive assessments this is often tested by asking the patient to name objects and carry out a written command.

Dyspraxia: difficulty coordinating or performing purposeful movements and gestures in the absence of motor or sensory impairments. In cognitive assessments this is often tested by asking the patient to draw a clock face or two intersecting pentagons.

Echolalia: repeating words spoken by another person, parrot-fashion.

Echopraxia: repeating the actions of another person.

Egodystonic: a thought that is experienced as troublesome and unwanted by the person experiencing it, who therefore tries to resist it. Obsessional thoughts are egodystonic.

Egosyntonic: a thought that is not experienced as unwanted or resisted.

Electroconvulsive therapy: treatment, usually for depression, that involves provoking seizures using controlled doses of electrical current applied through electrodes attached to the head (Chapter 37).

Expressed emotion (EE): the amount of critical and hostile comments and emotional over-involvement displayed in relationships, typically within the family. A high level of EE in the home has been associated with a worse prognosis in people with schizophrenia.

Extrapyramidal symptoms: side-effects of antipsychotic medication; includes Parkinsonian symptoms such as tremor, bradykinesia (slowness of movement) and akathisia (restlessness).

Flight of ideas: speech in which there is an abnormal connection between statements (see Chapter 2).

Flooding: type of behavioural therapy in which the patient is rapidly exposed to an anxiety-producing stimulus (Chapter 33).

Folie du pourquoi: the irresistible habit of seeking explanations for commonplace facts by asking endless questions (see Chapter 12).

Formal thought disorder: the patient's speech indicates that the links between consecutive thoughts are not meaningful; includes loosening of association.

Free association: the process in psychoanalysis whereby the patient is invited to say whatever comes into his or her mind.

Functional disorder: a psychiatric disorder in which there is no known physical cause (opposite of organic disorder).

Grandiosity: the patient's behaviour and speech indicate a belief that he or she is superior to others.

Habit reversal training: used in Tourette's syndrome, aims to increase awareness of tics and develop a competing response to them (e.g. relaxation).

Habituation: the decrease in anxiety that occurs with prolonged exposure to a situation that is initially anxiety-provoking (Chapter 33).

Hallucination: a perception in the absence of an external stimulus which is experienced as true and as coming from the outside world.

Hoarding: the acquisition of, and difficulty discarding, items that appear worthless to others. Occurs in OCD and also in people without a psychiatric disorder.

Hypochondriasis: a preoccupation with health that is regarded as excessive by an observer. The ideas may be overvalued (exaggerated in degree or importance) or fully delusional.

Ideas of reference: thoughts that other people are looking at or talking about the patient, not held with full delusional intensity.

Illusion: distortion of a normal perception (e.g. interpreting a curtain cord as a snake).

Incongruous affect: emotion expressed by a patient differs markedly from that which might be expected in the situation (e.g. bright, happy affect while describing a painful bereavement).

Insight: the patient's understanding of his or her condition, its cause and the patient's willingness to accept treatment.

Learning theory: the theoretical basis for behavioural therapy, that people will be more likely to repeat actions that are associated with rewards (see operant conditioning).

Loosening of associations: speech in which there is no discernable link between statements (see Chapter 2).

Makaton: a communication system of signs and gestures used by some people with severe learning disabilities.

Mannerism: goal-directed, understandable movement (e.g. saluting).

Modelling: learning a behaviour by copying (e.g. people may be more likely to drink heavily if exposed regularly to a heavy drinking environment).

Mood: how a person is feeling in themselves; in the mental state the subjective mood (how the patient describes his or her feeling) and objective mood (the interviewer's assessment).

Morbid: a thought or feeling that is held with such intensity and is so preoccupying that it causes significant distress (e.g. morbid fear of fatness in eating disorders, morbid jealousy). The term may encompass delusions, obsessions and overvalued ideas.

Motivational interviewing: client-centred counselling that facilitates change by exploring ambivalence to that change; it is used to encourage establishment of healthy eating in eating disorders and to promote abstinence in substance use disorders.

Negative symptoms (of schizophrenia): symptoms characterized by the loss of normal functions, including lack of motivation, decreased thoughts and speech, and social withdrawal.

Neologism: a made-up word (e.g. headshoe to mean hat); a second-rank symptom of schizophrenia.

Neuroleptic malignant syndrome: potentially fatal complication of antipsychotic treatment, involving hyperpyrexia, autonomic instability, confusion and increased muscle tone and raised serum creatine phosphokinase.

Neurosis: mental distress in which the ability to distinguish between symptoms originating from the patient's own mind and external reality is retained; includes most depressive and anxiety disorders.

Obsession: recurrent thoughts, feelings, images or impulses which are intrusive, persistent, senseless, and/or unwelcome but are recognized as the patient's own.

Onomatomania: a compulsion that involves the desire to utter a socially unacceptable or inappropriate word (see Chapter 12).

Operant conditioning: the basic process by which an individual's behaviour is shaped by reinforcement or punishment, for example, alcohol consumption may be maintained by the rewards (reinforcement) of associated social life and pleasant feelings of relaxation, and by punishment (unpleasant side-effects) if a dependent drinker stops.

Organic disorder: psychiatric disorder with an identifiable physical cause (e.g. drug use, physical illness).

Orientation: awareness of the current day, date, time and year (orientation to time), location (orientation to place) and personal details, such as name and age (orientation to person).

Overvalued idea: an acceptable, comprehensible idea pursued by the patient beyond the bounds of reason and to an extent that causes distress to the patient or those around him or her.

Panic attack: discrete period of intense fear, impending doom or discomfort, accompanied by characteristic somatic symptoms (see Chapter 11).

Perseveration: repeating words or topics.

Phobia: fear or anxiety that is out of proportion to the situation, cannot be reasoned or explained away, and leads to avoidance behaviour.

Positive symptoms: the symptoms of schizophrenia characterized by abnormal thoughts and perceptions (i.e. hallucinations and delusions).

Premorbid personality: a description of the patient's character and attitudes before he or she became unwell (e.g. personality [whether sociable, short-tempered], hobbies and interests), which is given in the psychiatric history (see Chapter 1).

Pressure of speech: speech in which rate and volume are increased; it is usually difficult to interrupt.

Projection: a defence mechanism that involves attributing one's own feelings about something to others.

Pseudo-hallucination: perception in the absence of an external stimulus, experienced in internal space (i.e. inside one's head), with preserved insight.

Pseudo-seizure: a seizure generated by the person deliberately or through subconscious processes rather than due to electrical activity in the brain.

Psychiatric Intensive Care Unit (PICU): psychiatric inpatient ward with extra security, and higher staff/patient ratio, designed to manage patients who require additional security during their admission, usually due to risk of violence or absconding.

Psychomotor agitation: an increase in overall motor activity; occurs in mania.

Psychomotor retardation: a decrease in overall motor activity; a sign of more severe depression.

Psychosis: severe mental disturbance characterized by a loss of contact with external reality. Delusions, hallucinations and disorganized thinking are often present.

Rapport: the interviewer's assessment of the warmth of relationship developed with the patient during an interview; it encompasses the extent of engagement and how forthcoming the patient was with information.

Rate of speech: the speed that a person speaks; usually increased in mania and often decreased in depression.

Reciprocal inhibition: a technique in behavioural therapy which links desensitization with a response incompatible with anxiety (e.g. relaxation, eating).

Rehabilitation psychiatry: branch of psychiatry concerned with recovery after serious psychiatric illness; there is usually a focus on psychological and social recovery.

Ritual: an action that has a 'magical' quality and is culturally sanctioned. This is not a psychiatric symptom but could potentially be confused with one by someone unfamiliar with the culture of the person performing the ritual.

Rumination: persistent preoccupation.

Somatic passivity: a delusion that an outside force is able to control one's bodily functions (e.g. generate sensations of heat or pain).

Somatization: the experience of psychological distress as actual physical symptoms, often pain.

Splitting: a defence mechanism that involves separating in one's mind the positive and negative qualities of self and others, so people are perceived as all good or all bad.

Stereotypy: repetitive, purposeless movements (e.g. rocking in people with severe learning disability).

Suicide: intentional self-inflicted death.

Systematic desensitization: graded exposure to a hierarchy of anxiety-producing situations.

Tardive dyskinesia: movements most often affecting the mouth, lips and tongue (e.g. rolling the tongue or licking the lips). They are usually the result of long-term administration of typical antipsychotics.

Thought block: a. subjective experience that thoughts suddenly disappear (see Chapter 2).

Thought broadcasting: a delusional belief that one's thoughts are available to others; this may include the belief that they are being broadcast to everyone around, or that they are known to specific people by a process similar to telepathy.

Thought echo: an auditory hallucination in which the patient hears his own thoughts spoken out loud.

Thought insertion: the patient experiences thoughts as being alien and not his or her own, and therefore believes that they have been inserted by an external force.

Thought withdrawal: a delusional belief that the patient's thoughts are removed from his or her head by an external force.

Tic: a local and habitual twitching, especially in the face.

Transference: term given to an unconscious process in which a patient re-experiences strong emotions from early important relationships in his/her relationship with a therapist.

Index

abstinence, 42–43
abuse, 15
  children, 15, 23, 44–45
  learning disabilities, 51
  sexual, 8, 34–35, 36–37, 44
  substance *see* substance abuse/misuse
acamprosate, 42–43
acceptance, grief reaction, 27
accidental harm, 15
acute intermittent porphyria (AIP), 64–65
acute intoxication, 32–33, 42–43
acute stress disorders (ASD), 26
Addison's disease, 32, 65, 78
adjustment disorder (AD), 12–13, 26–27, 60
adolescence, 13, 29, 48–49
Adults with Incapacity (Scotland) Act (2000), 85, 88
advance decision, 85
advance statements, 88
advocacy for patients, 83, 88
affect *see* mood
agoraphobia, 23, 28–29, 44–45
AIDS *see* HIV/AIDS
akathisia, 75
alcohol, 8–9, 15, 42–43, 65, 69
  adolescence, 49
  crime, 84
  cultural differences, 52–53
  delirium, 68–69
  depression, 23
  personality disorder, 34–35
  social exclusion, 54–55
  suicide, 16
alcoholic dementia, 42–43, 71
altruistic suicide, 17
Alzheimer' disease, 51, 65, 70–71
amisulpiride, 74
amitryptiline, 76
amnesic disorders, 64–65
  alcohol, 42–43
  substance abuse, 42–43
amok, 52–53
amphetamines, 25, 40–41
amyloid cascade hypothesis, 71
anankastic personality disorder, 30–31, 34–35
'Angel dust', 40–41
anhedonia, 22–23, 37, 61, 67
anomic suicide, 16–17
anorexia nervosa, 32–33, 49, 52–53
  compulsions and obsessions, 30–31
  suicide, 17
antiadrenergic drugs, 74–75, 76–77
anticholinergic drugs, 20, 74–75, 76–77
anticipatory fear, 29
anticonvulsants, 25
antidepressants, 22–23, 36, 61, 76–77
  anxiety, 28
  breastfeeding, 57
  bulimia nervosa, 33
  DSH, 17
  OCD, 31
  personality disorders, 35
  PTSD, 27
  schizophrenia, 21
antidopaminergic drugs, 74–75
antihistaminergic drugs, 74–75
antimanic agents, 78
antipsychotics (neuroleptics), 10, 36, 74–75
  adolescence, 49
  atypical, 20–21, 25, 49, 74–75
  bipolar affective disorder, 24–25

children, 46
  OCD, 31
  schizophrenia, 20–21
  typical, 20–21, 25, 49, 74–75
antisocial behaviour in children, 44–45
antisocial personality disorder, 34–35, 49, 86–87
  crime, 85
  suicide and DSH, 16–17
anxiety, 10–11, 13, 28–29 72–73
  adolescence, 48–49
  bipolar affective disorder, 25
  children, 44–45
  depression, 22–23
  pregnancy, 56–57
  stress, 26–27
anxiolytics, 28, 31, 57
appearance (in mental state exam), 10–11
approved mental health professional (AMHP), 86–87
approved mental practitioner (AMP), 88
approved social worker (ASW), 86–87, 90–91
aripiprazole, 74
arithmomania, 30
Asperger's syndrome, 46–47
aspirin, 70–71, 77
assertive outreach teams (AOTs), 82–83
asylum seekers, 54–55
ataque de nervios, 52–53
atomoxetine, 46
attention-deficit hyperactivity disorder (ADHD), 25, 46–47, 49, 65
autism, 46–47, 49, 50–51, 65
autoimmune inflammatory disorders, 64–65
automatic negative thoughts, 72
automatism, 85
aversion therapy, 42–43
avoidant personality disorder, 34–35
axes (DSM-IV-TR), 12–13

Bamford Review, 85, 90
Beck's cognitive triad, 22
behaviour, 13, 60–61
  adolescence, 48–49
  children, 44–45, 46–47
  learning disabilities, 51
  MSE, 10–11
behaviour therapy (BT), 44–45, 72–73
  bipolar affective disorder, 24–25
benzamides, 74
benzodiazepines (BDZs), 20, 36, 43, 69, 75, 78–79
  generalized anxiety disorder, 29
  misuse, 30, 40–41
bereavement, 8, 26–27, 45
  cultural differences, 52–53
bestiality, 36–37
beta-blockers, 28, 36, 75
bipolar affective disorder (BAD), 18, 24–25, 31
bipolar I disorder, 24–25
bipolar II disorder, 24–25
body dysmorphic disorder (BDD), 31
Body Mass Index (BMI), 32–33
borderline personality disorder, 34–35, 72–73
  suicide and DSH, 16–17
brain damage, 50–51
'brain fag', 52–53
breastfeeding, 57, 78
brief psychodynamic psychotherapy (BPT), 72–73
bulimia nervosa, 32–33, 49, 52–53, 76–77
bullying, 45
buprenorphine, 41
buproprion, 46

busiprone, 29
butyrophenones, 74

CAGE questions, 42–43
candidiasis, 67
cannabis, 40–41, 48–49
  schizophrenia, 18–19, 20–21
Capgras syndrome, 38
carbamazepine, 24–25, 57, 78
carbohydrate deficient transferrin (CDT), 43
care coordinator, 82–83
care plans, 14–15
Care Programme Approach (CPA), 20–21, 82–83
catatonic schizophrenia, 18–19
cathinone, 40–41
cerebrovascular accident (CVA; stroke), 58–59, 61, 62–63, 71
childbirth, 8–9, 25, 56–57
  depression, 32–33
children, 13, 44–45, 46–47
  abuse, 15, 23, 44–45
  personality disorders, 34–35, 44–45
  risk assessment, 15
chlordiazepoxide, 69, 79
chlorpromazine, 74
chronic fatigue syndrome, 52–53, 61
citalopram, 63, 76
classification, 12–13
clinical examination preparation, 92–93
  case studies, 99–101, 104–106
  EMQs, 96–98, 103
  OSCEs, 92–93, 94–95
clomipramine, 29, 30–31
clonidine, 46, 65
clopenthixol, 74
clozapine, 20, 65, 74–75
cocaine, 25, 39, 40–41
cognitive assessment, 10–11
cognitive behavioural therapy (CBT), 72–73
  adolescence, 49
  children, 45
  depression, 22–23, 59
  eating disorders, 32–33
  OCD, 31
  panic disorders, 28–29
  personality disorders, 34–35
  schizophrenia, 20–21
  stress reactions, 26–27
cognitive disorders, 13, 19, 63, 68–69
community care, 82–83, 87
  risk assessment, 14–15
  substance abuse, 41
Community Care Act (1991), 83
Community Health In-Reach Teams, 55
Community Mental Health Care Teams (CMHCTs), 82–83
Community Psychiatric Nurses (CPNs), 20, 82-3
compulsions, 30–31
compulsory treatment, 86–87, 88–89, 90–91
Compulsory Treatment Orders, 88–89
computed tomography (CT) scans, 69, 71
  schizophrenia, 19, 20–21
conduct (behavioural) disorders
  adolescence, 48–49
  children, 44–45, 46–47
confidentiality, 14–15
confusional states (delirium), 60–61, 68–69
consent, 87, 89, 91
  ECT, 80–1, 89, 91
consciousness, 10–11, 68–69
controlled drinking, 42–43

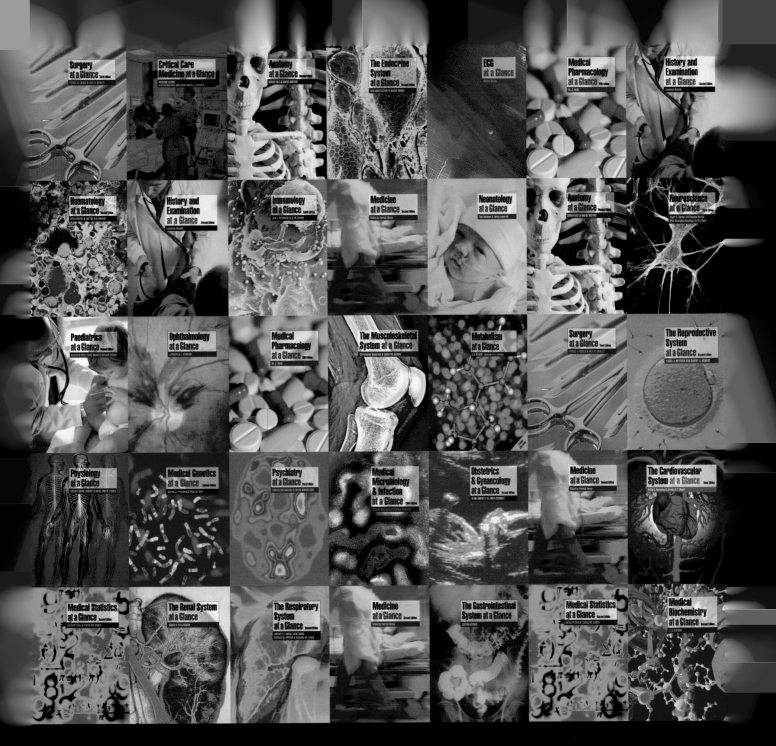

The at a Glance series

Popular double-page spread format • Coverage of core knowledge
Full-colour throughout • Self-assessment to test your knowledge • Expert authors

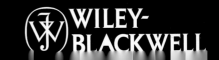

WILEY-
BLACKWELL

www.blackwellmedstudent.com

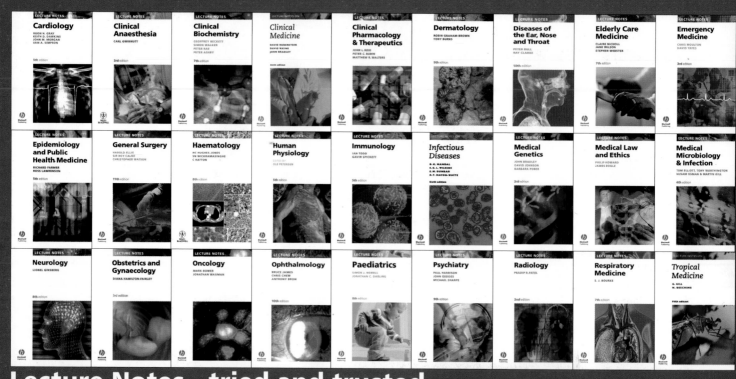
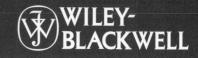

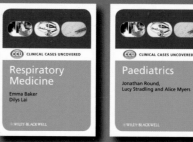
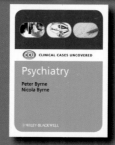
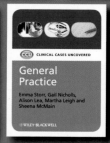
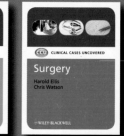
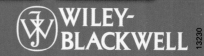